Workbook for

Laboratory and Diagnostic Testing in Ambulatory Care: A Guide for Health Care Professionals

Fourth Edition

Marti Garrels, MSA, MT (ASCP), CMA (AAMA)
Medical Assisting Program Consultant
Retired Medical Assisting Program Director
Lake Washington Institute of Technology
Kirkland, Washington

ELSEVIER

ELSEVIER

3251 Riverport Lane
St. Louis, Missouri 63043

WORKBOOK FOR LABORATORY AND DIAGNOSTIC TESTING IN AMBULATORY CARE: A GUIDE FOR HEALTH CARE PROFESSIONALS, FOURTH EDITION

ISBN: 978-0-323-53224-2

Notices

Knowledge and best practice in this field are constantly changing. As new research and experience broaden our understanding, changes in research methods, professional practices, or medical treatment may become necessary.

  Practitioners and researchers must always rely on their own experience and knowledge in evaluating and using any information, methods, compounds, or experiments described herein. In using such information or methods they should be mindful of their own safety and the safety of others, including parties for whom they have a professional responsibility.

  With respect to any drug or pharmaceutical products identified, readers are advised to check the most current information provided (i) on procedures featured or (ii) by the manufacturer of each product to be administered, to verify the recommended dose or formula, the method and duration of administration, and contraindications. It is the responsibility of practitioners, relying on their own experience and knowledge of their patients, to make diagnoses, to determine dosages and the best treatment for each individual patient, and to take all appropriate safety precautions.

  To the fullest extent of the law, neither the Publisher nor the authors, contributors, or editors, assume any liability for any injury and/or damage to persons or property as a matter of products liability, negligence or otherwise, or from any use or operation of any methods, products, instructions, or ideas contained in the material herein.

Content Strategist: Kristin R. Wilhelm
Content Development Manager: Lisa P. Newton
Content Development Specialist: Erin Garner
Publishing Services Manager: Shereen Jameel
Project Manager: Radhika Sivalingam
Cover Designer: Muthukumaran Thangaraj

Printed in the United States of America

Last digit is the print number: 9   8   7   6   5   4   3

Working together to grow libraries in developing countries

www.elsevier.com • www.bookaid.org

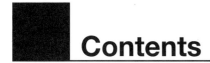

Contents

Copyright © 2019 Elsevier, Inc. All Rights Reserved.

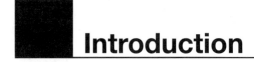

Introduction

This workbook is designed to build mastery over the highly technical and fascinating field of laboratory medicine. Each workbook chapter is organized into five sections: terminology exercises, review questions from: fundamental concepts, procedures, and advanced concepts, followed by: check-off procedure sheets for all the procedures presented in the chapter, and behavioral check-off sheets in the chapters that deal with patient interactions. The completed workbook exercises and check-off procedure sheets fulfill all the competency objectives listed at the beginning of each chapter in the textbook.

The appendix of the workbook contains laboratory maintenance logs, report forms, quality control logs, patient logs, a sample health screening assessment form, and a professionalism evaluation form. These forms provide the necessary documentation needed to prove laboratory quality assurance, safety compliance, and proper logging of test results.

TIPS FOR MASTERING EACH CHAPTER

Terminology Exercises

Before reading each chapter, you should become familiar with the technical terms related to the subject. The matching exercises in this workbook can be very helpful for learning the terms. In the textbook, each keyterm is set in blue bold type and defined in the context of the chapters to reinforce and build further understanding. There are also TEACH Student Handouts on the Evolve website (http://evolve.elsevier.com/Garrels/laboratory) for you to fill in the structured notes on your own or during the classroom lectures.

Basic Concepts, Procedures, Advanced Concepts—Review Questions and Labeling

The questions, pictures, and diagrams found in these three sections in the textbook and the workbook fulfill the stated objectives for each chapter. The workbook questions are designed to follow the textbook. You are encouraged to use the textbook alongside the workbook for visual reinforcement and as a reference for finding data from the tables and flow charts. The advanced concepts sections contain more complex critical thinking exercises as well as referencing detailed laboratory test information in Chapters 3 through 10. Your course instructor may choose to assign any or all of these advanced concept sections, depending on the time frame of the course.

Check-off Procedure Sheets

These outcome-based procedure sheets are found at the end of each workbook chapter. You are encouraged to locate the corresponding procedure box in the textbook, which provides pictures of the various steps involved in each procedure. For interested students, video presentations for many of the procedures are also located on the Evolve website. The procedures fall into two categories: *Skill Procedures* (e.g., using a microscope, instructing patients, collecting specimens, staining slides, and performing ECGs and spirometry) and *Analytical Testing Procedures* (e.g., urinalysis, hemoglobin, glucose, HIV, and strep tests), in which you follow a test procedure through the preanalytical, analytical, and postanalytical phases to obtain reliable test results. In both cases, it is very important that you read, perform, and be "checked off" of each step on the sheet as satisfactory or unsatisfactory. The steps marked with an asterisk (*) are critical to demonstrate and pass the competency. The *Skill Procedures* generally are performed with the instructor verifying each step. The *Analytical Testing Procedures* may be performed with a laboratory partner verifying the steps leading up to the test result. The instructor then verifies the final test result and the proper documentation of the test result to fulfill the required measurable outcome. *Behavioral Procedure* Check-off sheets have been added to this fourth edition in the chapters where patient interaction takes place:

- Chapter 3 – Instructing a Patient in Proper Urine Collection,
- Chapter 4 – Role-Playing Blood Collection Procedures With a Variety of Patients,
- Chapter 9 – Role-Playing Blood Collection With a Non-English Speaking Patient,
- Chapter 11 – Instructing a Patient How to Perform a Proper Spirometry Test.

USING THE WORKBOOK TO SET UP A CLINICAL CLIA-WAIVED LABORATORY

The chapter procedure sheets and all the quality assurance forms provided in the appendix may also be used to set up and monitor a CLIA-waived laboratory. The appendix forms are also available on the student Evolve website.

1 Introduction to the Laboratory and Safety Training

INTRODUCTION TO LABORATORY - VOCABULARY REVIEW

Match each definition with the correct term.

_____ 1. Most of the population will test within a range of similar results when testing an analyte

_____ 2. Laboratory orders indicating what tests are to be done

_____ 3. A steady state of internal chemical and physical balance

_____ 4. The substance being tested, such as glucose or cholesterol, in a body specimen

_____ 5. A test result indicating a threat to a patient's health

_____ 6. The patient's willingness to follow the treatment plan and take an active role in his or her own health care

_____ 7. Tests that provide simple, unvarying results and require a minimal amount of judgment and interpretation

_____ 8. Clotting ability of blood

_____ 9. A facility or an area within a medical setting in which materials or specimens from the human body are examined or analyzed

_____ 10. The inability to regulate blood sugar levels

_____ 11. Long-lasting, debilitating conditions

_____ 12. Disease-causing microorganisms

_____ 13. Outpatient health care setting in which patients are not bedridden

A. diabetes mellitus
B. homeostasis
C. reference range
D. pathogens
E. compliance
F. CLIA-waived tests
G. chronic disorders
H. analyte
I. critical value
J. ambulatory care
K. requisitions
L. coagulation
M. clinical laboratory

Identify the Following Acronyms

14. POCT _____

15. CBC _____

16. POL _____

FUNDAMENTAL CONCEPTS

Overview of the Laboratory

17. List the three reasons a physician would prescribe a laboratory test.

_____

_____

_____

18. List the three ways a specimen is analyzed.

_____

_____

_____

19. List the three types of medical laboratories.

_____

_____

_____

20. Give three reasons why a physician would want a test performed in the office and three reasons the specimen would be tested at an outside reference or hospital laboratory.

Advantages of In-Office Testing	Advantages of Out-of-Office Testing

21. List three examples of professional credentials (or titles) obtained by individuals who perform laboratory tests based on their educational degree or certification (see Table 1.1 in the textbook).

Doctorate: 8 or more years of education	Master's: 6 or more years of education	Bachelor's: 4 or more years of education	Associate Degree or Certificate: 1 to 2 years of education

22. Do a self-evaluation of your professionalism by using the form on page 3. Identify two areas you could improve by circling the description "objective" on the left column.

_____

_____

PROFESSIONAL EVALUATION FORM FOR THE LABORATORY CLASSROOM

Student: _____   Date: _____

Class: _____   Semester: _____

Number of Tardies: _____   Number of Hours Absent: _____

Objective	Very Satisfactory 3	Satisfactory 2	Unsatisfactory 1	Comments
Exhibits professional written communication (e.g., appearance, language, grammar)				
Uses the class materials appropriately (e.g., equipment, supplies, computers, cleanup)				
Provides instructor with all necessary information in a timely and organized manner (e.g., meets due dates, make-ups turned in within a week)				
Adheres to specific course policies (e.g., make-up guidelines, skill check-offs, externship guidelines)				
Projects a positive attitude and motivation (e.g., seen during lectures and labs)				
Displays professional verbal communication at all times (e.g., respectful, tactful)				
Maintains confidentiality of all personal interactions at all times (see rules of confidentiality in handbook)				
Projects professional work ethics (e.g., responsible, accountable, independent, full use of laboratory time: practice, study, computer)				
Cooperates with fellow students (e.g., team projects, skill practice, study groups)				
Displays responsible attendance behavior (e.g., arriving on time, calling in if detained or absent, prepared for next class session)				
Dresses appropriately (see handbook)				

Additional Comments:

_____

_____

_____   _____

Student Signature   Instructor

Chapter **1 Introduction to the Laboratory and Safety Training**

23. From the reference laboratory requisition form (see Fig. 1.7 in the textbook), write the first three laboratory tests listed in the following categories for blood, and provide the procedure code and blood collection container.

Test Category	First Three Listed Laboratory Tests (see Requisition)	CPT Code (see Column on the Left of Each Test)	Specimen Container (see Column on the Right of Each Test)
Hematology tests			
Chemistry tests			
Serology/immunology tests			

24. Give the metric unit and abbreviation for each basic unit of measurement.

Measurement	Metric Unit	Abbreviation
Weight		
Length		
Volume (capacity)		

25. Give the metric prefix and abbreviation for each of the following.

Fractions	Prefix	Abbreviation
1/10, or 0.1		
1/100, or 0.01		
1/1000, or 0.001		
1/1,000,000, or 0.000001		

26. All laboratory supplies have temperature storage directions on them. Where would a lab supply be stored if it had the following temperature ranges?

Store at 15° to 30°C _____

Store at 0° C _____

Store at 4° to 8°C _____

27. Give the military times for the following Greenwich times (see Table 1.4 in the textbook).

3:00 pm _____

8:35 am _____

9:15 pm _____

Noon _____

4

CAAHEP XII.P.1 Comply with: a. safety signs, b. symbols, c. labels

Match each definition with the correct term.

_____ 28. A documented plan provided by a facility to eliminate or minimize occupational exposure to bloodborne pathogens

_____ 29. Danger related to the exposure to toxic, unstable, explosive, or flammable materials

_____ 30. A means of transporting an infectious agent or pathogen from the infected individual to another by air, food, hand-to-hand contact, insects, or body fluids

_____ 31. The assumption that the blood or body fluid containing blood from any patient or test kit could be infectious

_____ 32. A disease that is spread within a health care facility

_____ 33. Federal law protecting employees' right to know about the dangers of the hazardous chemicals they may be exposed to under normal working conditions

_____ 34. Through the skin

_____ 35. An area that has been in contact with materials or environmental surfaces where infectious organisms may reside

_____ 36. Specialized clothing or equipment worn by an employee for protection against infectious materials

_____ 37. Efforts and research toward isolating and removing bloodborne pathogens from the workplace

_____ 38. Danger related to exposure to infectious and bloodborne pathogens

_____ 39. Dangers related to electricity, fire, weather emergencies, bomb threats, and accidental injuries

_____ 40. Policies that are recorded, monitored, and evaluated to protect employees from exposure to the pathogens in blood or body fluids

_____ 41. Putting on clothing or equipment as a barrier to a hazard

_____ 42. CDC recommendations for infection control in health facilities

A. chemical hazard
B. Standard Precautions
C. health care–associated infection (HCAI)
D. exposure control plan
E. percutaneous
F. work practice controls
G. Universal Precautions
H. donning personal protective equipment
I. transmission
J. physical hazards
K. engineering controls
L. personal protective equipment
M. hazard communication standard
N. contaminated
O. biohazards

Identify the Following Acronyms

43. Identify the following government safety regulatory agencies by their acronyms:

OSHA _____

HHS _____

CDC _____

Safety Training

CAAHEP COMPETENCIES: III.P.1., III.P.2., XII.P.4. XII.P5, VI.P.9.
ABHES COMPETENCIES: 9.a., 9.g.

44. List three ways that pathogens (infectious organisms) are transmitted.

_____

_____

_____

45. List three methods to sanitize hands. (Hint: Each uses a different cleanser.)

_____

_____

_____

46. Label the following personal protective equipment. (Hint: See Procedure 1.1.)

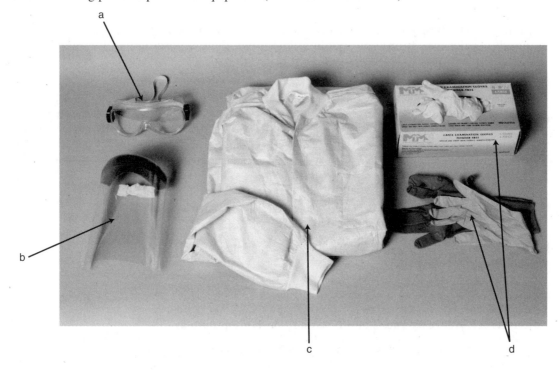

47. In which of the following disposal containers would contaminated gloves be disposed: wastebasket, biohazard waste container, or biohazard sharps container?

_____

48. List the three major bloodborne pathogens. (Hint: All are viral.)

_____

_____

_____

49. List two additional viruses that have emerged and are transmitted via contaminated blood.

_____

_____

50. Identify the following acronyms related to infections and to the bloodborne pathogen standard.

HCAIs _____

OPIM _____

PPE _____

PEP _____

51. Identify the following acronyms related to chemical hazard training.

SDS _____

NFPA _____

HMIS _____

52. List three safety rules (work practice controls) that must be observed in the laboratory and explain why.

_____

_____

_____

53. Use the Internet to locate and identify any OSHA or CDC updates on laboratory safety.

_____

Laboratory Safety Checklist

CAAHEP VI.P.9 Perform an inventory with documentation,

XII.P,2 Demonstrate the proper use of: a. eyewash equipment, b. fire extinguisher, c. sharps disposal containers

XII.P.5 Evaluate the work environment to identify unsafe working conditions.

Tour the laboratory with the following safety checklist and perform the bloodborne pathogen training posttest after the tour.

Item	Located
Physical safety	
First-aid kit	
Fire extinguisher	
Evacuation routes	
Fire	
Tornado	
Other (bomb threat)	
Chemical safety items	
Eyewash station	
Safety Data Sheets (SDS)	
Caustic spill kit (if needed)	
Acid spill kit (if needed)	
Hazardous labels	
Biological safety items	
Bleach disinfectant	
Biohazard spill kit	
Sharps container	
Biohazard container	
Hand sanitizing stations	
Safety devices on needles and lancets	
Personal protective equipment	
Gloves	
Eye goggles and face shields	
Laboratory coat/gown, liquid impenetrable	
Documentation resources	
SDS/safety manual	
Maintenance logs	
Quality control and patient logs	
Laboratory procedure manual	

OSHA Bloodborne Pathogen Quiz

1. A laboratory worker exposed to potentially infectious materials on the job may request a vaccine for which blood-borne disease?
   A. HIV
   B. syphilis
   C. hepatitis B
   D. brucellosis

2. Which of the following materials could contain bloodborne pathogens?
   A. bloody saliva
   B. semen
   C. vaginal secretions
   D. all of the above

3. If gloves are worn when cleaning up an accident site, washing the hands afterward is not necessary.
   A. true
   B. false

4. Bloodborne pathogens may enter the system through:
   A. open cuts
   B. skin abrasions
   C. dermatitis
   D. mucous membranes
   E. all of the above

5. All body fluids should be treated as infectious, and direct skin contact with them should be avoided.
   A. true
   B. false

6. Eating, drinking, and smoking should never take place in a laboratory or other area where potential exposure to bloodborne pathogens exists.
   A. true
   B. false

7. What should be done *first* after an exposure incident?
   A. file an exposure report
   B. wash the exposed area
   C. find out if the patient is infected
   D. consult a physician

8. Waste that is dripping blood must be placed in containers that are color coded or clearly labeled "biohazard."
   A. true
   B. false

9. A freshly diluted 10% solution of 1 part bleach to 9 parts water provides a strong enough solution to decontaminate most surfaces, tools, and equipment effectively.
   A. true
   B. false

10. How can puncture wounds from contaminated needles be avoided?
    A. discard used disposable needles in the appropriate container
    B. do *not* recap used needles (use safety activated devices)
    C. practice using safety devices before using on patients
    D. all of the above

11. **CAAHEP XII.P.4 Participate in a mock exposure event with documentation of specific steps.** Locate the Blood and Body Fluid Exposure Report Form in this workbook's Appendix Chapter 1. Given a mock exposure incident, fill out all five pages of the report form. Example: You were withdrawing a needle from a patient with hepatitis C, and you accidentally scraped your hand that was holding the gauze and it started to bleed. After you washed it thoroughly and reported it to your supervisor, you are asked to fill out the form. Fill out the form completely with what you think happened.

Procedure 1.1: Proper Use of Personal Protective Equipment
CAAHEP COMPETENCIES:
III.P.2.Select appropriate barrier/personal protective equipment (PPE)
III.P.3. Perform handwashing
ABHES COMPETENCIES: 9.a.

Person evaluated _____ Date _____

Evaluated by _____ Score _____

Outcome goal	Demonstrate the proper use of personal protective equipment
Conditions	Given the following supplies: hand sanitizer nonpowdered, nonlatex gloves fluid-impenetrable gowns or lab coats with cuffs at the wrists face masks and goggles, or full face shield (if the procedure to be performed has the potential for splashing)
Standards	Required time: 10 minutes Performance time: _____ Total possible points = _____ Points earned = _____

Evaluation Rubric Codes:
S = Satisfactory, meets standard. **U** = Unsatisfactory, fails to meet standard.

Preparation	Scores	
	S	U
1. Before donning (putting on) PPE, remember to perform the hand sanitizing appropriately.		

Procedure	Scores	
	S	U
2. Follow the proper sequence for donning PPE.		
a. Put on the gown.		
b. Don any face protectors.		
c. Don disposable, nonsterile, nonpowdered, nonlatex, well-fitting gloves.		
d. Extend the gloves over the gown cuffs.		
3. Keep gloved hands away from the face. Remove gloves if they become torn, and perform hand hygiene before donning new gloves. Avoid touching other surfaces and items not involved in the testing process. The outside of the front of the gown is considered contaminated. The "clean" areas of the gown and gloves are on the inside and the back of the gown.		
4. Sequence for removing PPE:		
a. Properly remove gloves as follows:		
Remove one glove by grasping the outside with the other gloved hand and pulling it off (glove-to-glove contact).		
Wad up the removed glove in the gloved hand. Slip an ungloved finger under the other cuff (skin to skin) and fold it over until you can grasp the inside area of the second glove and fold it over the contaminated glove.		
Pull off the second glove inside-out with the first glove still inside.		
If the gloves have visible blood or body fluid on them, dispose of them in a biohazard waste receptacle.		
b. Remove the face shield by pulling it off from behind the head or from the ear attachments forward.		
c. Remove the gown carefully by avoiding the contaminated areas (outside of the gown front and sleeves)		
NOTE: If fluid-impenetrable lab coats are reused in the lab, close the lab coat with the clean inside protected before hanging it up. The gown must not leave the lab area.		

Follow-up	Scores	
	S	U
5. Perform hand hygiene (hand wash or hand rub) immediately after removing PPE.		
Total Points per Column		

2 Regulations, Microscope Setup, and Quality Assurance

VOCABULARY REVIEW

Match each definition with the correct term.

_____ 1. Tests that produce a result measured as a number

_____ 2. A substance or ingredient used in a laboratory test to detect, measure, examine, or produce a reaction

_____ 3. An overall process to aid in improving the reliability, efficiency, and quality of laboratory test results

_____ 4. Materials with known values of the substance measured that help the laboratory achieve accurate and reliable testing by checking if the test system is working

_____ 5. A visible result indicating the presence of a substance a test is designed to detect

_____ 6. Proving competency by testing a specimen from an outside accreditation agency

_____ 7. Tests that look for the presence or absence of a substance

_____ 8. A process in which known samples (controls) are routinely tested to establish the reliability, accuracy, and precision of a specific test system

_____ 9. All components of a test that are packaged together

_____ 10. A built-in positive control to prove the device or test kit is working

_____ 11. The awareness and prevention of both the physical and the procedural risks that may bring about an injury or legal action against the practice

_____ 12. A pattern of narrow and wide bars and spaces; each pattern is encoded with its own particular meaning

_____ 13. When both accuracy and precision are accomplished

_____ 14. Liquid positive and negative controls that are tested the same way as the liquid patient specimen

_____ 15. Ability to produce the same test result each time a test is performed (results are seen clustered together on a target)

_____ 16. The average test result of a series of controls

_____ 17. A statistical term describing the amount of variation from the mean in a dataset

_____ 18. When controls consistently fall within the two standard deviations of the mean (results are seen within the center of a target)

_____ 19. Used to plot the daily results of the control samples

_____ 20. A result indicating the absence of the substance that the test is designed to detect

_____ 21. Any substance in a sample, other than the one being measured or detected, whose presence affects the result of the test being performed

_____ 22. When the internal control area on a qualitative test shows no reaction during the testing process

A. reactive/positive
B. quality assurance
C. qualitative
D. quality control
E. kit
F. quantitative
G. reagent
H. proficiency testing
I. controls
J. accuracy
K. Levey-Jennings chart
L. medical office risk management
M. bar codes
N. reliability
O. standard deviation
P. precision
Q. internal control
R. external controls
S. mean
T. invalid test
U. nonreactive/negative
V. interfering substance

13

Government Acronyms Worksheet

As you write the words for each government acronym or abbreviation, note its relationship to the various divisions of government and its effect on ambulatory laboratories.

Federal departments	HHS (Oversees the 4 divisions below) =				Department of Labor	
Divisions within the department	OCR = Office of Civil Rights	CMS =	FDA =	CDC =	OSHA =	
Laws or regulations affecting laboratories	HIPAA: OCR enforces privacy standards	HIPAA: CMS enforces insurance portability		**Infection control:**	**Infection control, blood:**	
		CLIA: CMS administers laboratory certifications	CLIA: FDA classifies laboratory test complexity	CDC recommends Standard Precautions for all infectious diseases	OSHA regulates **BBPS** =	Hazard communication standard; OSHA regulates chemical hazards
Additional acronyms and abbreviations	HIPAA =	CLIA =	CoW =		PPE =	MSDS =
		QA =			OPIM =	HMIS =
	PHI =	QC =	PPM =		PEP =	NFPA =
Additional notes						

CLIA Government Regulations

23. What is the purpose of the **C**linical **L**aboratory **I**mprovement **A**mendments of 1988 (CLIA 1988) Act, and how does it benefit the patient?

_____

_____

24. What are the three categories of testing under CLIA, and under which category is physician-performed microscopy listed?

_____

_____

_____

25. Review Table 2.1 in the textbook, which lists most of the CLIA-waived tests available. Locate three tests in each category, and list their corresponding procedure codes on the following chart:

Test Category	Physician Office Tests	Procedure Code (CPT; 5-digit code)
Hematology tests		
Blood chemistry tests		
Serology/immunology tests		
Microbiology tests (only two)		

26. From the provider-performed microscopy procedure in Table 2.2 in the textbook, write the procedure codes for each of the following:

a. Wet mounts, including preparations of vaginal, cervical, or skin specimens _____

b. Urinalysis (microscopic only) _____

c. All potassium hydroxide preparations _____

Chapter **2** **Regulations, Microscope Setup, and Quality Assurance**

27. Label the microscope, and perform the microscopic procedure at the end of the chapter.

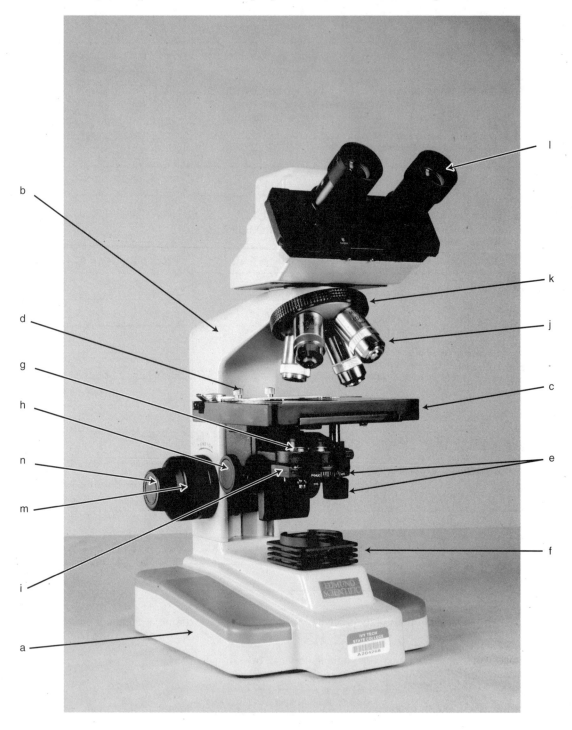

28. List the structures under each of the functional areas of the microscope.

Foundational	Illuminating	Magnifying
a.	f.	j.
b.	g.	k.
c.	h.	l.
d.	i.	
e.		

GOOD LABORATORY PRACTICES

CAAHEP COMPETENCIES: II.P.2.,
ABHES COMPETENCIES: 10.a, 10.c.,

Quality Assurance

29. Quality assurance oversees what three areas (or phases) of good laboratory practices? Specimen collection takes place during what phase of good laboratory practices?

_____

_____

_____

30. What is the difference between qualitative tests and quantitative tests, and how does it affect quality control?

_____

_____

_____

31. Explain the relationship between accuracy, precision, and reliability when plotting the results of standard controls.

_____

_____

_____

_____

32. Locate and list the following CDC Tips, Reminders, and Resources from Fig. 2.9 in the textbook:

READY? List four tips to **"Check"** and two tips to **"Perform."**

Check _____

Check _____

Check _____

Check _____

Perform _____

Perform _____

SET? List a tip to **"Check"** and a tip to **"Wear."**

Check _____

Wear _____

TEST? List two tips to **"Follow"** and two tips to **"Report."**

Follow _____

Follow _____

Report _____

Report _____

33. A. Plot the 4 weeks of daily glucose control results on the four blank Levey-Jennings graphs below, and answer questions B & C for each week's graph:

CAAHEP COMPETENCIES: II.P.3.
ABHES COMPETENCIES: 10.a

A. Plot the numerical results for each day on its weekly graph below.

WEEK 1: day 1 = 103, day 2 = 100, day 3 = 98, day 4 = 112, day 5 = 105, day 6 = 99

B. Circle whether week 1 is experiencing a *trend*, a *shift*, a *random error*, or is *out of control*.

C. How would you correct the quality control issue seen in WEEK 1? _____

B. Week 1 glucose control results show: _____

C. Possible way to correct: _____

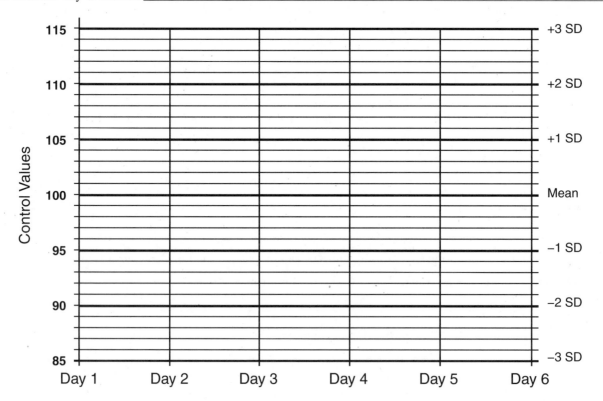

A. Plot the numerical results for each day on its weekly graph below.

WEEK 2: day 1 = 94, day 2 = 92, day 3 = 93, day 4 = 108, day 5 = 109, day 6 = 107

B. Circle if Week 2 glucose control results a *trend,* a *shift,* a *random error,* or is *out of control.*

C. Possible way to correct: _____

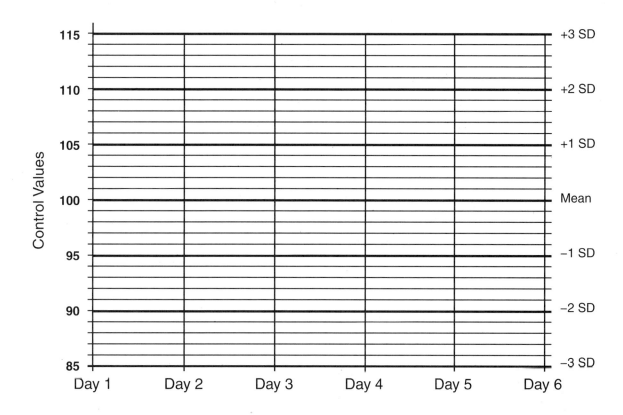

Chapter **2** **Regulations, Microscope Setup, and Quality Assurance**

A. Plot the numerical results for each day on its weekly graph below.

WEEK 3: day 1 = 90, day 2 = 95, day 3 = 100, day 4 = 105, day 5 = 108, day 6 = 110

B. Circle if Week 3 glucose control results are experiencing a *trend*, a *shift*, a *random error*, or is *out of control*.

C. Possible way to correct: _____

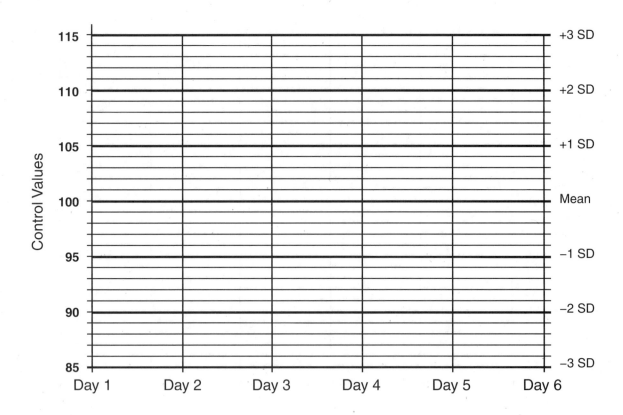

A. Plot the numerical results for each day on its weekly graph below.

WEEK 4: day 1 = 100, day 2 = 103, day 3 = 98, day 4 = 112, day 5 = 115, day 6 = 113

B. Circle if Week 4 glucose control results are experiencing a *trend*, a *shift*, a *random error*, or is *out of control*.

C. Possible way to correct: _____

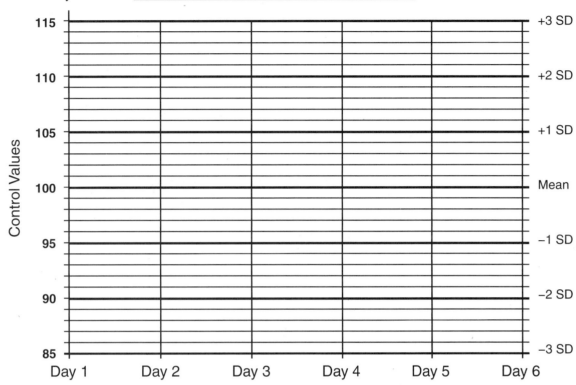

HIPAA Privacy Rule, Risk Management, Electronic Medical Records, and Bar Coding

34. Are laboratory personnel allowed to give an interested party a patient's test results? Why or why not? Base your answer on the Health Insurance Portability and Accountability Act (HIPAA) and risk management principles of avoiding financial and legal consequences.

_____

_____

_____

_____

35. What is the most important use of bar codes in the medical laboratory?

_____

_____

Chapter **2** **Regulations, Microscope Setup, and Quality Assurance**

10 STEPS TOWARD GOOD LABORATORY PRACTICE

1. Upon receiving a **new test kit** (which contains all the components of a test that are packaged):
   a. **Make sure it is a CLIA-waived test** (this information may be printed on the box, printed in the package insert, in a letter to the manufacturer from HHS, or found on the Web at https://www.accessdata.fda.gov/scripts/cdrh/cfdocs/cfCLIA/seardh.cfm or https://www.cms.gov/clia.
   b. **Keep the manufacturer's product insert** for the test in use in a procedure manual. Always use the product insert for the kit currently in use. Read the product insert each time a kit is opened to check for **changes in procedures** or **quality control.**

2. Follow the manufacturer's instructions regarding **proper specimen collection** and handling:
   a. **Use appropriate collection containers.**(i.e., proper blood-collecting tubes and/or test kit devices, urine collection containers, microbiology swabs, etc.)
   b. **Store specimens at the proper temperature and time interval** (i.e., room temperature and/or refrigerated).

3. **Properly identify the patient.**
   a. Does the name on the **test requisition** (or prescription) match the patient's name?
   b. Does the name on the **patient's chart** match the name on the patient's identification?
   c. **If more than one patient is present with the same first and last name:** Look for possible gender differences, social security number, patient identification number, birth dates, different middle name, and relevance of the test to the patient's history.)

4. **Inform the patient** of any **test preparation,** such as fasting, clean catch urine, special diet, etc.

5. **Label the patient's specimen** for testing with an identifier unique to each patient.

6. **Read the product insert** completely prior to performing a test.
   a. **Become familiar with the test procedure.**
   b. **Study each step** and perform them in the proper order.
   c. **Know the time required** for performing the test and achieving the optimal result.
   d. **Have all of the required reagents and equipment ready** before performing the test.
   e. **Perform quality control testing** whenever a new test kit is opened prior to testing patient samples. For automated waived testing, quality control procedures must be consistent with manufacturer's recommendations and are performed on each instrument used at least once on each day of patient testing. **Control testing results must be recorded on a quality control log.**
   f. Be able to **recognize when the test is finished**—e.g., will there be a blue plus-or-minus sign against a white background?

7. **Follow the storage requirement for the test kit**—e.g., stored away from direct light, temperature requirements, open container expiration dates, etc. Write the expiration date on the kit.

8. **Do not mix components of different kits!**

9. **Record the patient's test results** in the proper place, such as the patient's chart and the laboratory test log, but *not* on unidentified sticky notes or pieces of scrap paper that can be misplaced.
   a. **Record the results** according to the instructions in the manufacturer's product insert.
   b. **If it's a qualitative test, spell out positive/negative** or **pos/neg** because the symbolic representations can be altered (the – can be altered to a +).
   c. **Include the name of the test, the date the test was performed, and the initials of the testing personnel** in the test record. Include the calendar year in the date.
   d. **If the same test is performed on a patient multiple times** in one day, include the time of each test.

10. **Perform any instrument maintenance** as directed by the manufacturer.

Refer to the two forms needed to set up a laboratory procedure manual at the end of this workbook chapter: Qualitative Test Template, and Quantitative Test Template.

Procedure 2.1: Using a Microscope

Person evaluated _____   Date _____

Evaluated by _____   Score _____

Outcome goal	To bring a stained slide into focus from low power to high dry power and then focus on oil immersion
Conditions	Given a microscope; lens paper; a stained slide; immersion oil; and soft, lint-free tissue
Standards	Time = 15 minutes Accuracy = each step on check sheet is completed, and an image is focused on oil immersion for evaluator check-off before cleanup

Evaluation Rubric Codes:
S = Satisfactory, meets standard   **U** = Unsatisfactory, fails to meet standard

Total possible points = _____   Points earned = _____

NOTE: Steps marked with an asterisk (*) are critical to achieve required competency.

Preparation	Scores	
	S	U
1. Carry the microscope with two hands, uncover, and adjust for cleaning.		
- Place one hand under the base, and with the other, grasp the arm of the scope.		
2. Turn the coarse focus until the stage and objectives are farthest apart.		
3. Clean the ocular and all objective lenses with lens paper (clean oil lens last).		
4. Turn the nosepiece to low power (shortest tube).		
- Do not push on objective tubes; use the nosepiece to turn.		
5. Adjust light settings.		
- Bring the condenser all the way up for a stained specimen.		
- Open the iris diaphragm all the way with the lever.		
6. Position a stained slide over the light source.		
- Place the slide with stained side up into the mechanical holder clamp.		
- By using the mechanical control, move the slide until the stained area is above the light.		
7. Adjust the ocular lens to line up with the eyes.		

Procedure	Scores	
	S	U
Low-Power Focus		
8. While looking through the oculars, turn the coarse adjustment until color starts to appear, and then turn slowly to bring the image into coarse focus.		
- Always start with the low-power objective to avoid breaking the slide.		
- Move the slide back and forth slightly with the mechanical controls to detect movement.		

	S	U
9. Move hand to fine-focus adjustment, and turn one way and then the other until the image becomes clear.		
- Make sure both eyes are seeing a clear image; if not, adjust the oculars by turning their individual focus controls.		
10. Move the slide to a place of interest in the center of the visual field, and then turn the nosepiece to high power.		
High-Power Focus		
11. Refocus the image by turning the fine adjustment one way and then the other until color is seen; then slowly bring in a clear image.		
- Do not use coarse adjustment because it would make too drastic a change and possibly break the slide. If the fine adjustment cannot focus, go back to low power, and start again with the coarse and fine-focus adjustments.		
- Move the slide so that something interesting is in the middle.		
Oil Immersion Preparation and Focus		
12. Turn the nosepiece halfway between high power and the oil immersion objective.		
13. Place a drop of oil directly on the slide where the condenser light is shining.		
14. Carefully turn the nosepiece until the oil immersion lens dips into the oil and snaps into place.		
*15. While looking into the oculars, move the small fine-focus adjustment back and forth until the image pops into view.		
When image is in view, obtain instructor verification. _____		
- Scan the slide to see cells or organisms.		
- Use one hand on the mechanical control to move the slide, and use the other hand on the fine focus to make continual adjustments.		

	Scores	
Follow-up: Cleanup and Microscope Maintenance	S	U
16. Turn off the light, and turn the nosepiece back to the low-power objective.		
- Turn the coarse-focus knob to maximize the distance between the lens and the stage.		
- Remove the slide, and clean the stage with soft, lint-free tissue.		
- Clean oil off the slide with the tissue or xylene.		
17. With lens paper, clean off the ocular lenses and objective lenses; the oil immersion lens is always the last to be cleaned.		
*18. Cover the microscope with a dust-proof cover, and store in a clean, protected area.		
Total Points per Column		

*The instructor or supervisor verifies a successfully focused result. This step is critical to achieve required competency.

Analytical Testing

Qualitative Test: _____

Person evaluated _____   Date _____

Evaluated by _____   Score _____

Outcome goal	
Conditions	Supplies required:
Standards	Required time = _____ minutes
	Performance time = _____
	Total possible points = _____ Points earned = _____
Evaluation Rubric Codes: **S** = Satisfactory, meets standard **U** = Unsatisfactory, fails to meet standard	
NOTE: Steps marked with an asterisk (*) are critical to achieve required competency.	

Preparation: Preanalytical Phase	Scores	
	S	U
A. Test information		
- Kit method: _____		
- Manufacturer: _____		
- Proper storage (e.g., temperature, light): _____		
- Lot number of kit: _____		
- Expiration date: _____		
- Package insert or test flow chart available: _____ yes _____ no		
B. Personal protective equipment		
C. Specimen information		

Procedure: Analytical Phase	Scores	
	S	U
D. Performed/observed qualitative quality control		
- External liquid controls: Positive _____ Negative _____		
- Internal control:		
E. Performed patient test		
1.		
2.		
3.		
4.		
REACTIVE/POSITIVE seen as:		
NONREACTIVE/NEGATIVE seen as:		
INVALID seen as:		
*Accurate Results _____ Instructor Confirmation _____		

Follow-up: Postanalytical Phase	Scores	
	S	U
*F. Proper documentation		
1. On control/patient log: _____ yes _____ no		
2. Documented on patient chart (see later in section).		
3. Identified "critical values" and took appropriate steps to notify physician.		
EXPECTED VALUES FOR ANALYTE:		
G. Proper disposal and disinfection		
1. Disposed of all sharps in biohazard sharps containers.		
2. Disposed of all other regulated medical waste in biohazard bags.	1.	
3. Disinfected test area and instruments according to OSHA guidelines.	3.	
4. Sanitized hands after removing gloves.	4.	
Total Points per Column		

Patient Name: _____

Patient Chart Entry: (Include when, what, why, any additional information, and the signature of the person charting.)

_____

_____

_____

Analytical Testing

Quantitative Test: _____

Person evaluated _____   Date _____

Evaluated by _____   Score _____

Outcome goal		
Conditions		
Standards	Required time = _____ minutes	
	Performance time = _____	
	Total possible points = _____	Points earned = _____

Evaluation Rubric Codes:
S = Satisfactory, meets standard   **U** = Unsatisfactory, fails to meet standard

NOTE: Steps marked with an asterisk (*) are critical to achieve required competency.

Preparation: Preanalytical Phase	Scores	
	S	**U**
A. Test information		
- Kit or instrument method: _____		
- Manufacturer: _____		
- Proper storage (e.g., temperature, light): _____		
- Lot number of kit or supplies: _____		
- Expiration date: _____		
- Package insert or test flow chart available: _____ yes _____ no		
B. Specimen information		
- Type of specimen and preparation (e.g., fasting, first morning): _____ _____		
- Specimen container or testing device: _____		
- Amount of specimen: _____		
C. Personal protective equipment		
D. Assembled all the above, sanitized hands, and applied PPE		

Procedure: Analytical Phase	Scores	
	S	**U**
E. Performed/observed quality control for A or B		
Quantitative testing controls		
- Calibration check: _____		
- Control levels: Normal _____ High _____ Low _____		

F. Performed patient test		
Followed proper steps (see test flow chart and list):		
1.		
2.		
3.		
4.		
5.		
6.		
7.		
8.		
9.		
10.		
*Accurate Results _____ Instructor Confirmation _____		

Follow-up: Postanalytical Phase	Scores	
	S	U
*G. Proper documentation		
1. On control log: _____ yes _____ no		
2. On patient log: _____ yes _____ no		
3. Documented on patient chart (see next page).		
4. Identified "critical values" and took appropriate steps to notify physician.		
EXPECTED VALUES FOR ANALYTE:		
H. Proper disposal and disinfection		
1. Disposed of all sharps into biohazard sharps containers.		
2. Disposed of all other regulated medical waste into biohazard bags.		
3. Disinfected test area and instruments according to OSHA guidelines.		
4. Sanitized hands after removing gloves.		
Total Points per Column		

Patient Name: _____

Patient Chart Entry: (Include when, what, why, any additional information, and the signature of the person charting.)

_____

_____

_____

3 Urinalysis

VOCABULARY REVIEW

Match the function with the correct anatomic term.

_____ 1. Functional unit of the kidney

_____ 2. Part of the nephron that contains the glomerulus and glomerular capsule

_____ 3. Structure in the renal corpuscle made up of tangled blood capillaries in which the hydrostatic pressure in the capillaries pushes substances through the capillary pores

_____ 4. Cup-shaped structure surrounding the glomerulus that collects the glomerular filtrate

_____ 5. Tube that carries urine from the bladder to the outside of the body.

_____ 6. Two muscular tubes 10 to 12 inches long that carry urine formed in the kidneys to the urinary bladder

_____ 7. Hollow, muscular organ that holds urine until it is expelled

_____ 8. Tube that carries urine outside the body

_____ 9. Referring to the area behind the peritoneal cavity

_____ 10. Parts of the nephron composed of proximal convoluted tubules, the nephron loop (loop of Henle), and distal convoluted tubules

A. urethral meatus
B. glomerulus
C. glomerular (Bowman's) capsule
D. urinary bladder
E. renal tubules
F. nephron
G. renal corpuscle
H. ureters
I. retroperitoneal
J. urethra

Match each term related to urinalysis with the correct definition. (Note: Definitions and terms are continued on the next page.)

_____ 11. Caused by treatment or diagnostic procedures

_____ 12. Substance that easily loses electrons

_____ 13. Intact red blood cells in the urine

_____ 14. Protein found in the urine of patients with multiple myeloma

_____ 15. Painful urination

_____ 16. Red cells breaking open and releasing hemoglobin

_____ 17. Expelling of urine, also referred to as voiding and urination

_____ 18. The weight of urine compared with the weight of an equal volume of water; measures the amount of dissolved substances in urine

_____ 19. No urine flow

_____ 20. Sugars (especially glucose) in the urine

_____ 21. To break open

_____ 22. Decreased urine volume

A. electrolyte
B. renal threshold level
C. oliguria
D. bilirubin
E. anuria
F. dysuria
G. nocturia
H. diuresis
I. porphyrin
J. glycosuria
K. reducing substances
L. ketonuria
M. hematuria
N. lyse
O. hemolysis
P. proteinuria
Q. pyuria
R. iatrogenic
S. lipiduria
T. casts

_____ 23. Ketones in the urine

_____ 24. Excessive urination at night

_____ 25. Intermediate substance in the formation of heme (part of hemoglobin)

_____ 26. Element or compound that forms ions when dissolved and is able to conduct electricity

_____ 27. Proteins in the urine

_____ 28. Lipids in the urine

_____ 29. Increase in the volume of urine output

_____ 30. Waste product from the breakdown of hemoglobin

_____ 31. White blood cells in the urine

_____ 32. Elements excreted in the urine in the shape of the renal tubules and ducts

_____ 33. Blood reabsorption limit of a substance and the point at which the substance is then excreted in the urine

_____ 34. Scale that measures the level of acidity or alkalinity of a solution

U. micturition
V. pH
W. specific gravity
X. Bence Jones protein

FUNDAMENTAL CONCEPTS

Anatomy of the Urinary System

35. Label the structures of the urinary system.

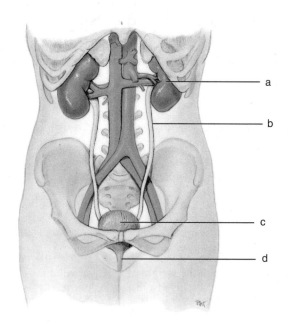

a

b

c

d

36. Label the structures of the kidney.

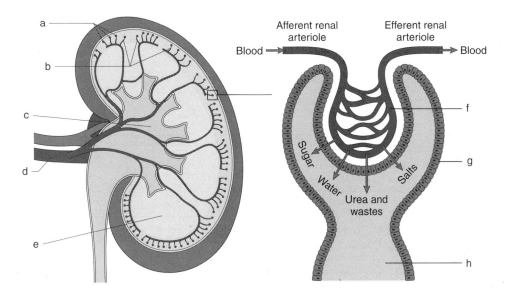

37. List the four general functions of the urinary system.

1. _____

2. _____

3. _____

4. _____

38. Describe the location of the kidneys in the body.

_____

_____

39. List the functions of the nephron.

_____

_____

40. Name the two structural components of the nephron.

_____   _____

_____

41. List and describe the two components of the renal corpuscle.

_____

_____   _____

_____

42. Describe the three steps of urine formation.

_____

_____

_____

43. Explain the term *renal threshold*.

_____

_____

44. Discuss the importance of a urinalysis.

_____

_____

45. Name the three parts of a urinalysis.

_____

_____

_____

Urine Specimen Collection

46. Discuss the advantages of the first morning specimen.

_____

_____

_____

_____

47. Give three general requirements for all types of urine collection methods.

_____

_____

_____

48. Discuss the proper handling and discarding of urine specimens.

_____

_____

49. When educating a female patient about the steps involved in preparing for midstream clean-catch urine, why must the patient understand the importance of wiping from front to back?

_____

_____

_____

CLINICAL LABORATORY IMPROVEMENT AMENDMENT (CLIA)–WAIVED URINALYSIS TESTS

Physical Urinalysis

50. Name the tests that are part of the physical urinalysis.

_____

_____

51. List the terms used to describe the appearance of urine.

_____

_____

52. Give the range of normal color for urine.

_____

_____

53. In what condition can urine have a sweet or fruity odor?

_____

_____

54. Discuss three abnormal urine colors and their causes.

_____

_____

_____

55. Describe the relevance of the specific gravity test in the urinalysis.

_____

_____

Chemical Urinalysis

56. Discuss the differences between qualitative, semiquantitative, and quantitative testing.

_____

_____

57. Label the urinalysis chemistry supplies (see Fig. 3.10 in the textbook).

A _____ B _____ C _____ D & E _____

58. Name the 10 urinalysis chemistry tests that are most frequently performed. (Hint: See the SG 10 urinalysis strips).

1. _____   6. _____
2. _____   7. _____
3. _____   8. _____
4. _____   9. _____
5. _____   10. _____

59. Discuss the reasons for the new method that tests for microalbumin.

_____

_____

_____

60. List three conditions that may cause blood to be found in urine.

_____

_____

_____

61. Explain why a first morning urine sample is recommended when testing for nitrites.

_____

_____

62. If the nitrite test is negative, could bacteria be present in the urine?

_____

_____

63. Name a confirmatory test that can be performed when a urine sample is positive for the bilirubin test.

_____

64. Describe the Clinitek instrument, including its advantages and disadvantages.

_____

_____

_____

65. List three guidelines related to urinalysis chemistry reagent strips.

_____

_____

_____

66. Describe the quality control methods available for urinalysis chemistry testing. (Hint: See question 57.)

_____

_____

67. You just ran the Chek-Stix positive control and recorded the results shown on the next page. Look at the expected results table for a positive control, located on the next page, and then circle the analyte that did **not** fall in its control range. Why do you suppose it did not record correctly? (Hint: Look at how the dipstick enters the urine specimen.)
   - Glucose—negative
   - Bilirubin—positive
   - Ketones—positive
   - Specific gravity—1.015
   - Blood—large
   - pH—8.5
   - Protein   100 mg/dL
   - Urobilinogen—3 mg/dL
   - Nitrate—positive
   - Leukocytes—moderate

Test	Expected Results With Bayer Reagent Strips and Tablets	
	Chek-Stix Positive Control	Chek-Stix Negative Control
Glucose	100-250 mg/dL	Negative
Bilirubin	Positive	Negative
Ketone	Positive	Negative
Specific gravity	1.000-1.015 (adjusted for pH)	1.010-1.025 (adjusted for pH)
Blood	Moderate, large	Negative
pH	≥8.0	6.0-7.0
Protein	Trace, 100 mg/dL (SI units: trace, 1.0 g/L)	Negative
Urobilinogen	≥2 mg/dL	0.2-1 mg/dL
Nitrite	Positive	Negative
Leukocytes	Trace, moderate	Negative
Microbumintest	Positive (by using 1:3 dilution of Chek-Stix positive control solution)	Negative
Acetest	Positive	Negative
Clinitest	250-750 mg/dL	Negative
Ictotest	Positive	Negative

68. Circle the patient results that are **not** in the normal reference range. (Note: Normal results would agree with the "Negative Control" column above.) What would be the probable cause for the abnormal urinalysis physical and chemical results, and what might the physician do next?
   - Dark yellow
   - Cloudy
   - Glucose—negative
   - Ketones—negative
   - Bilirubin—negative
   - Specific gravity—1.025
   - pH—7
   - Blood—2
   - Urobilinogen—0.2
   - Protein—moderate
   - Nitrite—positive
   - Leukocyte—moderate

_____

_____

_____

69. Circle the patient results that are abnormal compared with the urinalysis "normal" reference ranges (shown under "Negative Control" above). What is the probable cause for the abnormal urinalysis chemical results?
   - Glucose—2%
   - Ketones—moderate
   - Bilirubin—negative
   - Specific gravity—1.025
   - pH—6
   - Blood—negative
   - Urobilinogen—0.2
   - Protein—trace
   - Nitrite—negative
   - Leukocyte—negative

70. For the standardized urinalysis Kova system and the preparation of the microscopic examination, define the terms *sediment* and *supernatant* and state which of these is used in the microscopic examination of urine.

_____

_____

ADVANCED CONCEPTS: MICROSCOPIC URINALYSIS

71. Name four factors that can lead to cast formation.

_____

_____

_____

_____

72. Name the crystals that resemble envelopes (with an "X" appearance).

_____

_____

73. What parts of the microscopic urinalysis can be performed by a medical assistant (preanalytical, analytical, and/or postanalytical)?

_____

_____

74. Match the pictures of urine cells, casts, and crystals, and others with their microscopic drawings. (See Fig. 3-14, MICROSCOPIC URINALYSIS ATLAS in your textbook.)

Cells

Use these terms to identify the following illustrations: 1. red blood cells (RBCs), 2. white blood cells (WBCs), 3. squamous epithelial cells, and 4. renal tubular epithelial cells.

_____

_____

_____

_____

Casts

Use these terms to identify the following illustrations of casts on low power: 5. hyaline casts, 6. Granular casts, 7. RBC casts, 8. WBC casts, 9. Waxy cast

_____

_____

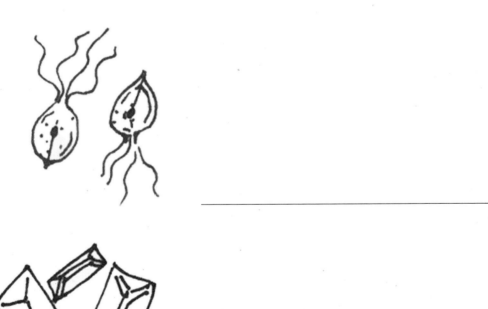

_____

_____

_____

Crystals and Other Forms

Use these terms to identify the following illustrations: calcium oxalate crystals, triple phosphate crystals, yeast, and *Trichomonas vaginalis*.

_____

_____

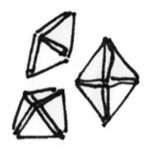

_____

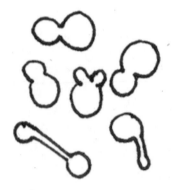

_____

BEHAVIORAL

Procedures 3-1, 2, and 3: Instructing Patients How to Collect Urine Specimens

Work in groups of three students each. Each student will play a different role in the first three instructional procedures (female clean-catch urine, male clean-catch urine, and 24-hour urine collection). When acting as the medical assistant giving instructions, sign the top line below and have two other students sign in with their respective roles (patient or evaluator).

Medical assisting student being evaluated _____

Student playing the role of the patient _____

Student evaluator: _____ (check off both the Behavioral and the Procedural sections based on your observations and then sign and date the forms)

CAAHEP AFFECTVE "BEHAVIORAL" COMPETENCY I.A.3.

COMPETENCY:	I.A.3. Show awareness of a patient's concerns related to procedure 3-2, Instructing a Female or Male Patient in Clean-Catch, or procedure 3-3, 24-Hour Urine Collection
OBJECTIVE(s):	Given the conditions, and provided the necessary supplies, the student will demonstrate awareness of patient concerns as they provide patient care in a role-play scenario for a student-partner.
TIME FRAME:	15 minutes
GRADING:	**PASS = 100% accuracy.** All steps must be completed as written for "**PASS.**" Students are permitted two (2) graded attempts. **Grading Instructions:** When step is performed as written, record a "✓" for "**PASS.**" When step is omitted and/or there is an error in written procedure, record instructor initials for "**FAIL.**" Procedure must be repeated.

STEP #	PROCEDURE (check the procedure you performed as a medical assistant student) ___ 3-1. Female clean-catch urine instructions ___ 3-2. Male clean-catch urine instructions ___ 3-3. 24-hour urine collection instructions	GRADED ATTEMPT 1		GRADED ATTEMPT 2	
		PASS	FAIL	PASS	FAIL
Example	Instructions to evaluator: Student **completes step** as written, record "✓" Student **omits step or performs it in error,** record initials	✓	ZH		
1.	Gathered supplies and reviewed the new or established patient's medical history form.				
2.	Correctly prepared the patient: ■ Greeted the patient, introduced self, escorted him/her to exam room, and verified name. ■ Made appropriate eye contact with the patient ■ Established a professional and empathetic atmosphere ■ Explained procedure to patient				
3.	Responded to patient concerns: ■ Showed empathy toward patient ■ Assured patient concerns are understood by repeating them and verifying them with patient ■ Explained procedure again to ensure patient understanding ■ Answered any questions from patient ■ Assured patient that procedure is necessary ■ Provided necessary follow-up contact information				

Evaluator signature _____ MA student signature _____

Date _____

Procedure 3-1: Instructing Female Patient How to Collect a Clean-Catch Urine Specimen—

Person evaluated _____   Date _____

Evaluated by _____

Outcome goal	Instruct a female patient regarding the correct procedure for midstream clean-catch specimen.
Conditions	Given the following - Sterile urine collection container and label - Antiseptic towelettes
Standards	Required time: 15 minutes Performance time: _____

Evaluation Rubric Codes:
S = Satisfactory, meets standard   **U** = Unsatisfactory, fails to meet standard

Total possible points = _____   Points earned = _____

NOTE: Steps marked with an asterisk (*) are critical to achieve required competency.

Preparation	Scores	
	S	**U**
1. Washed hands and gathered the appropriate equipment.		
2. Greeted and identified the patient.		

Procedure Instructions to Patient	Scores	
	S	**U**
3. Instructed patient to sanitize her hands and remove underwear.		
4. Instructed patient to spread apart the labia to expose the urinary opening.		
- Patient told to keep this area spread apart with the nondominant hand during the entire cleaning procedure.		
5. Instructed patient to take one antiseptic towelette and clean one side of the urinary opening from front to back, stressing the importance of the direction.		
- Patient told that cleaning in this direction will prevent anal organisms from being spread to the urinary opening.		
6. Instructed patient to take another antiseptic towelette and clean other side of the urinary opening from front to back, stressing the importance of the direction.		
7. Instructed patient to use a third antiseptic towelette to wipe from front to back directly across the urinary opening, stressing the importance of the direction.		
8. Instructed patient to continue to keep labia spread apart and to urinate a small amount (one-third of bladder volume) into the toilet, being careful not to touch the inside of the sterile container.		
- Patient told that the reason for urinating a small amount into the toilet is to flush away microorganisms that may be around the urinary opening.		
9. Instructed patient to collect the second part of the urine sample into the sterile container.		
- Student was able to state that this would collect the midstream portion of the urine specimen.		
10. Instructed patient to urinate the last portion of the urine into the toilet.		
11. Instructed patient to dry the area with a tissue.		

	Scores	
12. Instructed patient on the correct procedure after the specimen has been collected.		
- Instructed patient to cap the specimen carefully.		
- Instructed patient to place specimen in a certain area after collected in an office setting or to refrigerate if collected at home.		

	S	U
Follow-up		
13. After receiving specimen from patient, the sample was labeled correctly, and the requisition was completed if required.		
14. Washed hands.		
*15. Procedure was charted correctly.		
- Charted that female patient was given instructions for midstream clean-catch urine collection.		
- Charted reception of specimen from patient.		
Total Points per Column		

Patient Name: _____

Patient Chart Entry: (Include when, what, how, why, any additional information, and the signature of the person charting.)

_____

_____

_____

Procedure 3-2: Instructing Male Patients How to Collect a Clean-Catch Urine Specimen

Person evaluated _____   Date _____

Evaluated by _____

Outcome goal	Instruct a male patient in the correct procedure for midstream clean-catch specimen
Conditions	Given: - Sterile urine collection container and label - Antiseptic towelettes
Standards	Required time: 15 minutes Performance time: _____ Total possible points = _____ Points earned = _____

Evaluation Rubric Codes:
S = Satisfactory, meets standard   **U** = Unsatisfactory, fails to meet standard

Total possible points = _____   Points earned = _____

NOTE: Steps marked with an asterisk (*) are critical to achieve required competency.

Preparation	Scores	
	S	**U**
1. Washed hands and gathered the appropriate equipment.		
2. Greeted and identified the patient.		

Procedure	Scores	
	S	**U**
3. Instructed patient to sanitize his hands and remove underwear.		
4. If patient is uncircumsized, instructed the patient to retract the foreskin and hold it back during the entire procedure.		
5. Instructed the patient to clean the area around the penis opening by starting at the tip of the penis and cleaning downward using a separate antiseptic towelette for each side.		
6. Instructed patient to use a third antiseptic towelette to clean across the opening.		
*7. Instructed patient to urinate a small amount (one-third of bladder volume) into the toilet, being careful not to touch the inside of the sterile container.		
- Patient told that the reason for urinating a small amount into the toilet is to flush away microorganisms that may be around the urinary opening.		
8. Instructed patient to collect the second part of the urine sample into the sterile container.		
- Student was able to state that this would collect the midstream portion of the urine specimen.		
9. Instructed patient to urinate the last portion of the urine into the toilet.		
10. Instructed patient to dry the area with a tissue if needed.		

Follow-up	Scores	
	S	U
11. Instructed the patient on the correct procedure after the specimen has been collected.		
- Instructed the patient to carefully cap the specimen.		
- Instructed patient to place specimen in a certain area after collected in an office setting or to refrigerate if collected at home.		
12. After receiving the specimen from the patient, the sample was labeled correctly and requisition was completed if required.		
13. Washed hands.		
14. Procedure was charted correctly.		
- Charted that male patient was given instructions for midstream clean-catch urine collection.		
- Receiving of specimen from patient was charted.		
Total Points per Column		

Patient Name: _____

Patient Chart Entry: (Include when, what, how, why, any additional information, and the signature of the person charting.)

_____

_____

_____

Procedure 3-3: Instructing Patients How to Collect a 24-Hour Urine Specimen

Person evaluated _____   Date _____

Evaluated by _____

Outcome goal	To educate the patient on the correct instructions for collection of a 24-hour urine specimen
Conditions	Given: - Large urine container - Instructions sheet (see Fig. 3.6 and instructions in textbook) - Requisition
Standards	Required time: 15 minutes Performance time: _____

Evaluation Rubric Codes:
S = Satisfactory, meets standard   **U** = Unsatisfactory, fails to meet standard

Total possible points = _____   Points earned = _____

NOTE: Steps marked with an asterisk (*) are critical to achieve required competency.

Preparation	Scores	
	S	**U**
1. Washed hands and gathered the appropriate equipment.		
2. Greeted and identified the patient.		

Procedure	Scores	
	S	**U**
3. Instructed patient when arising on the first day of the 24-hour collection procedure to empty bladder into the toilet.		
- Instructed patient to record this time.		
4. Instructed the patient that all urine for 24 hours after that first voided specimen must be voided directly into the collection container.		
- Informed the patient to be sure to screw the lid on tightly each time and keep the container refrigerated.		
- Informed the patient that if at any time during the procedure some urine is not collected, the test will need to start again. Gave examples of this.		
5. Instructed the patient that on the second morning of the 24-hour period, the patient must arise at the same time as the first day and urinate directly into the container, keeping this sample.		
- Patient was instructed that the first morning specimen on the second day of the 24-hour period is the last sample collected and is the completion of the collection procedure.		
6. Instructed the patient that on the day the procedure is completed the container must be returned to the physician's office or to the laboratory.		

Follow-up	Scores	
	S	**U**
7. After the patient completed the procedure and returned the container, the patient was asked if any problems occurred during the collection procedure.		
8. Completed a laboratory requisition form for test ordered.		
9. Prepared the specimen to be transported to the laboratory that will perform the testing.		
*10. Charted the instructions and equipment supplied to the patient.		
- When patient returned with specimen, charted that the specimen was sent to the laboratory, documenting all necessary information concerning the specimen.		
Total Points per Column		

Patient Name: _____

Patient Chart Entry: (Include when, what, how, why, any additional information, and the signature of the person charting.)

_____

_____

_____

Procedure 3-4: Manual Chemical Reagent Strip Procedure

Person evaluated _____   Date _____

Evaluated by _____

Outcome goal	Perform a physical and chemical test on an unknown sample according to stated conditions and standards
Conditions	Given: - Reagent strips - Timing device - Reference chart - Requisition
Standards	Required time: 10 minutes Performance time: _____
Evaluation Rubric Codes: **S** = Satisfactory, meets standard Total possible points = _____	**U** = Unsatisfactory, fails to meet standard Points earned = _____
NOTE: Steps marked with an asterisk (*) are critical to achieve required competency.	

Preparation: Preanalytical Phase	Scores	
	S	**U**
A. Test information		
- Kit or instrument method: **Multistix 10 SG**		
- Manufacturer: **Bayer Corporation**		
- Proper storage (e.g., temperature, light): **room temperature, no direct sunlight**		
- Expiration date _____		
- Lot number _____		
- Package insert or test flow chart _____ yes _____ no		
B. Proper specimen		
- Special patient preparation (e.g., fasting, special diet, first morning specimen): **no special preparation**		
- Appropriate container: **clean container without preservatives**		
- Amount of specimen: **25 to 50 mL of well-mixed urine**		
C. Personal protective equipment: **gloves, gown, and biohazard container**		

Procedure: Analytical Phase	Scores	
	S	**U**
*D. Performed/observed quality control methods		
1. Semiquantitative liquid controls		
- Control levels: Normal _____ Abnormal _____		

*E. Performed patient test		
1. Hands were sanitized and equipment assembled.		
2. Urine was poured into a clear container or centrifuge tube.		
3. The color of the urine was determined.		
4. The clarity of the urine was determined.		
5. Strip was removed from the bottle, and the bottle was immediately closed. The pads on the strip were not touched, and the strip was held parallel to the chart.		
6. The pads were completely covered with urine. The pads were not immersed too long, which could cause the reagents to dissolve and leach out into the urine.		
7. After removing the strip from the urine, the strip was tapped against the side of the tube to remove excess urine.		
8. The color of each strip pad was read at a particular time and compared with the reference chart.		
*Accurate Results (see attached forms) Instructor Confirmation		

Follow-up: Postanalytical Phase	Scores	
	S	U
*F. Proper documentation		
1. On control log: _____ yes no _____		
2. On patient log: _____ yes no _____		
3. Documentation on patient chart forms on next page		
4. Identified critical values and took appropriate steps to notify physician.		

Analyte Expected Values

Glucose	Negative
Bilirubin	**Negative**
Ketone	**Negative**
Specific gravity	**1.005-1.030**
Blood	**Negative**
pH	**6.0-8.0**
Protein	**Negative/trace**
Urobilirubin	**Normal**
Nitrite	**Negative**
Leukocytes	**Negative**

G. Proper disposal and disinfection		
1. Disposed of strip into appropriate biohazard container.		
2. Poured the remaining urine down sink with stream of water and placed container in appropriate waste container.		

3. Disinfected test area and instruments according to OSHA guidelines.		
4. Sanitized hands after removing gloves.		
Total Points per Column		

Patient Name: _____

Patient Chart Entry: (Include when, what, how, why, any additional information, and the signature of the person charting.)

_____

_____

_____

Procedure 3-5: Clinitek Analyzer Method for Chemical Reagent Strip

Person evaluated _____   Date _____

Evaluated by _____

Outcome goal	Perform a physical and chemical test on an unknown sample according to stated conditions and standards
Conditions	Given: - Gloves - Multistix 10SG reagent strips or MultistixPro10SL strips - Absorbent paper - Clinitek analyzer
Standards	Required time: 5 minutes Performance time: _____

Evaluation Rubric Codes:
S = Satisfactory, meets standard   **U** = Unsatisfactory, fails to meet standard

Total possible points = _____   Points earned = _____

NOTE: Steps marked with an asterisk (*) are critical to achieve required competency.

Preparation: Preanalytical Phase	Scores	
	S	**U**
A. Test information		
- Kit or instrument method: **Multistix 10 SG and Clinitek instrument**		
- Manufacturer: **Bayer Corporation**		
- Proper storage (e.g., temperature, light): **room temperature, no direct sunlight**		
- Expiration date _____		
- Lot number _____		
- Package insert or test flow chart _____ yes _____ no		
B. Proper specimen		
- Special patient preparation (e.g., fasting, special diet, first morning specimen): **no special preparation**		
- Appropriate container: **clean container without preservatives**		
- Amount of specimen: **25 to 50 mL of well-mixed urine**		
C. Personal protective equipment: **gloves, gown, and biohazard container**		

Procedure: Analytical Phase	Scores	
	S	**U**
*D. Performed/observed quality control methods		
1. Semiquantitative liquid controls		
- Control levels: Normal (negative) _____ Abnormal (positive) _____		

*E. Performed patient test		
1. Mixed room-temperature urine sample and poured it into a conical tube before testing.		
2. Removed strip from bottle, closing bottle immediately. Did not touch the reagent pads.		
3. Followed instructions on the instrument monitor or the manufacturer's flow sheet. ■ Entered technician identification ■ Entered patient information ■ Before pressing the "start" command, had test strip ready to dip into the urine		
4. After pressing start, completed the following within 8 seconds: ■ **Dipped** the strip into the urine, ensuring all the pads were completely covered with urine, but did not immerse it too long ■ **Removed** excess urine from the strip by pulling the nonpad side of the strip along the edge of the container ■ **Blotted** the side of the strip against absorbent paper briefly ■ **Placed** the strip in the Clinitek tray, ensuring it was placed correctly		
5. **Note:** If the reagent strip was placed incorrectly, an error message appeared, and the tray pushed the sample out. The reagent strip was discarded, the instrument was reset, and a new reagent strip was used to run the test again.		
6. While the instrument was measuring timed reagent pads, the color and transparency of the urine specimen were keyed into the analyzer.		
7. When the test was complete, the analyzer displayed and printed the date, the time, the patient's name, the name of the person testing, the results of the 10 tests, the color, and a transparency.		
*Accurate Results (see attached forms or printed form) Instructor Confirmation _____		

	Scores	
Follow-up: Postanalytical Phase	**S**	**U**
*F. Proper documentation _____		
1. On control log: _____ yes _____ no		
2. On patient log: _____ yes _____ no		
3. Documentation on patient chart forms on next page		
4. Identified critical values and took appropriate steps to notify physician.		

Analyte Expected Values

Glucose	**Negative**
Bilirubin	**Negative**
Ketone	**Negative**
Specific gravity	**1.005-1.030**
Blood	**Negative**
pH	**6.0-8.0**
Protein	**Negative/trace**
Urobilirubin	**Normal**
Nitrite	**Negative**
Leukocytes	**Negative**

G. Proper disposal and disinfection		
1. Disposed of strip into appropriate biohazard containers.		
2. Disposed of all other regulated medical waste into biohazard bags.		
3. Disinfected test area and instruments according to OSHA guidelines.		
4. Sanitized hands after removing gloves.		
Total Points per Column		

Patient Name: _____

Patient Chart Entry: (Include when, what, how, why, any additional information, and the signature of the person charting.)

_____

_____

_____

Procedure 3-6: Clinitest Procedure for Reducing Substances Such as Sugars in the Urine

Person evaluated _____ Date _____

Evaluated by _____

Outcome goal	Perform a Clinitest test on an unknown sample
Conditions	Given: - Clinitest bottle of tablets - Clinitest tube - Tube of water with pipette - Urine sample with pipette - Clinitest reference chart
Standards	Required time: 15 minutes Performance time: _____

Evaluation Rubric Codes: _____

S = Satisfactory, meets standard **U** = Unsatisfactory, fails to meet standard

Total possible points = _____ Points earned = _____

NOTE: Steps marked with an asterisk (*) are critical to achieve required competency.

Preparation: Preanalytical Phase	Scores	
	S	U
A. Test information		
- Kit or instrument method: **Clinitest**		
- Manufacturer: **Bayer Corporation**		
- Proper storage (e.g., temperature, light): **room temperature with the lid tightly sealed; protect tablets from light, heat, and moisture**		
- Lot number of kit _____		
- Expiration date _____		
- Package insert available _____ yes _____ no		
B. Specimen information		
- Labeled urine specimen in clean container		
- Amount: **2 or 5 drops (according to directions)**		
C. Personal protective equipment: **gloves, sharps, and biohazard**		

Procedure: Analytical Phase	Scores	
	S	U
D. Performed/observed quality control		
1. Semiquantitative testing controls		
- Control levels: Normal _____ Abnormal _____		

E. Performed patient test		
1. Added 5 drops of urine to 10 drops of water in a Clinitest tube.		
2. Tapped the Clinitest tablet into the tube, which was placed in a rack because the boiling reaction that occurs is very hot.		
3. During the boiling reaction, the tube was observed for any color change.		
- The boiling reaction should be observed for the pass through effect, which results in color change occurring during the reaction and appears negative when the reaction is completed and results are determined.		
4. Shook the tube 15 seconds after the boiling had stopped to mix the contents.		
5. Compared color of the reaction with the Clinitest chart for the 5-drop method and recorded the results.		

*Accurate Results _____ Instructor Confirmation _____

	Scores	
Follow-up: Postanalytical Phase	**S**	**U**
*F. Proper documentation _____		
1. On control log: _____ yes _____ no		
2. On patient log: _____ yes _____ no		
3. Documentation on patient chart (see below)		
4. Identified critical values and took appropriate steps to notify physician. Expected values for analyte: **negative**		
G. Proper disposal and disinfection		
1. Disposed of all other regulated medical waste into biohazard bags.		
2. Disinfected test area and instruments according to OSHA guidelines.		
3. Sanitized hands after removing gloves.		
Total Points per Column		

Patient Name: _____

Patient Chart Entry: (Include when, how, what, why, any additional information, and the signature of the person charting.)

_____

_____

_____

Procedure 3-7: Procedure for the Preparation and the Microscopic Examination of Urine

Person evaluated _____   Date _____

Evaluated by _____

Outcome goal	To prepare a microscopic urinalysis slide, focus the slide on the microscope, and state the elements that can be found under low and high power.
Conditions	Given: - Gloves - Urine specimen - Kova equipment: cap, pipette - Sternheimer-Malbin stain - Test tube - Centrifuge - Microscope
Standards	Required time: 10 minutes Performance time: _____

Evaluation Rubric Codes:
S = Satisfactory, meets standard   **U** = Unsatisfactory, fails to meet standard

Total possible points = _____   Points earned = _____

NOTE: Steps marked with an asterisk (*) are critical to achieve required competency.

Preparation	Scores	
	S	U
1. Washed hands, applied gloves, and gathered the appropriate equipment.		
*2. Mixed the correctly identified room-temperature urine specimen.		
*3. Poured the urine sample to the "12 mark" in a urine centrifuge tube and capped the tube.		

Procedure	Scores	
	S	U
Performed procedure		
*4. Centrifuged the tube for 5 minutes at 1500 rpm.		
- Stated the definition of *sediment* and *supernatant*.		
*5. Carefully removed the spun tube from the centrifuge and removed the cap.		
*6. Carefully placed the Kova pipette into the bottom of the tube.		
- Hooked the clip on the top of the pipette over the outside of the tube.		
*7. Placed index finger on tip of the pipette and decanted off the supernatant by inverting the tube.		
- Stated the approximate amount of sediment that remained in the tube.		
8. Removed the pipette from the tube; added a drop of stain; and reinserted the pipette, squeezing gently to mix the urine sediment and stain.		
- Stated the purpose of using the stain.		

*9. Correctly transferred a drop of the urine sediment to a well in a Kova slide.		
- Did not overfill or underfill the well.		
*10. Allowed the Kova slide to sit for 1 minute.		
- Stated why the slide should sit.		
11. Stated who is qualified to perform a urine microscopic examination.		
12. Demonstrated the ability to focus a slide on the microscope.		
- Focused first with low power with the coarse adjustment.		
- Was able to fine focus with the fine adjustment knob.		
*13. Stated what elements are observed under low power.		
*14. Stated what elements are observed under high power.		

*Accurate Results _____ **Instructor Confirmation** _____ .

Follow-up: Postanalytical	Scores	
	S	U
Proper disposal and disinfection		
15. Demonstrated the proper procedure for cleaning, carrying, and storing the microscope.		
16. Correctly discarded the equipment in the appropriate containers.		
- Discarded the urine specimen in the appropriate manner.		
17. Removed and discarded gloves in the appropriate biohazard containers.		
18. Sanitized hands.		
19. Demonstrated an understanding of the process for calculating a urinalysis microscopic examination.		
Total Points per Column		

Patient Name: _____

Patient Chart Entry: (Include when, what, how, why, any additional information, and the signature of the person charting.)

_____

_____

_____

Form 1

Patient:

Doctor: DOB:

Date/Time Spec. Collected:

Date/Time Spec. Completed:

☐ VOID ☐ CC ☐ CATH ☐ TURBID ☐ HAZY ☐ CLEAR

TEST	REFERENCE	RESULT	TEST	REFERENCE	RESULT
Color	Yellow		Blood	Neg	
Char.	Clear		pH	5.0 - 8.0	
Glucose	Neg		Protein	Neg	
Bilirubin	Neg		Urobili	0.2 - 1.0 EU	
Ketone	Neg		Nitrite	Neg	
Sp. Gr	1,000 - 1,030		Leuk	Neg	

MICRO

TEST	REFERENCE	RESULT	TEST	REFERENCE	RESULT
WBC	0 - 5 HPF		Bact.	0 - 5	
RBC	0 - 3 HPF		Mucus	0	
Epith.	D		Casts	0	
Cryst.	0 - 3 HPF				

OTHER:

Form 2

Patient:

Doctor: DOB:

Date/Time Spec. Collected:

Date/Time Spec. Completed:

☐ VOID ☐ CC ☐ CATH ☐ TURBID ☐ HAZY ☐ CLEAR

TEST	REFERENCE	RESULT	TEST	REFERENCE	RESULT
Color	Yellow		Blood	Neg	
Char.	Clear		pH	5.0 - 8.0	
Glucose	Neg		Protein	Neg	
Bilirubin	Neg		Urobili	0.2 - 1.0 EU	
Ketone	Neg		Nitrite	Neg	
Sp. Gr	1,000 - 1,030		Leuk	Neg	

MICRO

TEST	REFERENCE	RESULT	TEST	REFERENCE	RESULT
WBC	0 - 5 HPF		Bact.	0 - 5	
RBC	0 - 3 HPF		Mucus	0	
Epith.	D		Casts	0	
Cryst.	0 - 3 HPF				

OTHER:

Form 3

Patient:

Doctor: DOB:

Date/Time Spec. Collected:

Date/Time Spec. Completed:

☐ VOID ☐ CC ☐ CATH ☐ TURBID ☐ HAZY ☐ CLEAR

TEST	REFERENCE	RESULT	TEST	REFERENCE	RESULT
Color	Yellow		Blood	Neg	
Char.	Clear		pH	5.0 - 8.0	
Glucose	Neg		Protein	Neg	
Bilirubin	Neg		Urobili	0.2 - 1.0 EU	
Ketone	Neg		Nitrite	Neg	
Sp. Gr	1,000 - 1,030		Leuk	Neg	

MICRO

TEST	REFERENCE	RESULT	TEST	REFERENCE	RESULT
WBC	0 - 5 HPF		Bact.	0 - 5	
RBC	0 - 3 HPF		Mucus	0	
Epith.	D		Casts	0	
Cryst.	0 - 3 HPF				

OTHER:

Form 1

Patient: \
Doctor: \
DOB: \
Date/Time Spec. Collected: \
Date/Time Spec. Completed:

	TEST	REFERENCE	RESULT	TEST	REFERENCE	RESULT		TEST	REFERENCE	RESULT
☐ VOID	Color	Yellow		Blood	Neg			WBC	0 - 5 HPF	
☐ CC	Char.	Clear		pH	5.0 - 8.0			RBC	0 - 3 HPF	
☐ CATH	Glucose	Neg		Protein	Neg		MICRO	Epith.	D	
☐ TURBID	Bilirubin	Neg		Urobili	0.2 - 1.0 EU			Cryst.	0 - 3 HPF	
☐ HAZY	Ketone	Neg		Nitrite	Neg			Bact.	0 - 5	
☐ CLEAR	Sp. Gr	1,000 - 1,030		Leuk	Neg			Mucus	0	
								Casts	0	
							OTHER:			

Form 2

Patient: \
Doctor: \
DOB: \
Date/Time Spec. Collected: \
Date/Time Spec. Completed:

	TEST	REFERENCE	RESULT	TEST	REFERENCE	RESULT		TEST	REFERENCE	RESULT
☐ VOID	Color	Yellow		Blood	Neg			WBC	0 - 5 HPF	
☐ CC	Char.	Clear		pH	5.0 - 8.0			RBC	0 - 3 HPF	
☐ CATH	Glucose	Neg		Protein	Neg		MICRO	Epith.	D	
☐ TURBID	Bilirubin	Neg		Urobili	0.2 - 1.0 EU			Cryst.	0 - 3 HPF	
☐ HAZY	Ketone	Neg		Nitrite	Neg			Bact.	0 - 5	
☐ CLEAR	Sp. Gr	1,000 - 1,030		Leuk	Neg			Mucus	0	
								Casts	0	
							OTHER:			

Form 3

Patient: \
Doctor: \
DOB: \
Date/Time Spec. Collected: \
Date/Time Spec. Completed:

	TEST	REFERENCE	RESULT	TEST	REFERENCE	RESULT		TEST	REFERENCE	RESULT
☐ VOID	Color	Yellow		Blood	Neg			WBC	0 - 5 HPF	
☐ CC	Char.	Clear		pH	5.0 - 8.0			RBC	0 - 3 HPF	
☐ CATH	Glucose	Neg		Protein	Neg		MICRO	Epith.	D	
☐ TURBID	Bilirubin	Neg		Urobili	0.2 - 1.0 EU			Cryst.	0 - 3 HPF	
☐ HAZY	Ketone	Neg		Nitrite	Neg			Bact.	0 - 5	
☐ CLEAR	Sp. Gr	1,000 - 1,030		Leuk	Neg			Mucus	0	
								Casts	0	
							OTHER:			

4 Blood Collection

VOCABULARY REVIEW

Match each term with the correct definition.

Fundamental Concept Terms

_____ 1. Area in front of the elbow

_____ 2. Blood vessels with a pulse that carry blood away from the heart

_____ 3. Microscopic blood vessels that contain a mixture of arterial and venous blood

_____ 4. Blood collection; derived from the Greek words *phlebo*, meaning vein, and *tomy*, meaning to cut

_____ 5. Blood vessels with valves that carry blood toward the heart

_____ 6. Gently touching and pressing down on an area to feel texture, size, and consistency

_____ 7. Fluid or semifluid substances found in the body

A. humors
B. palpating
C. arteries
D. capillaries
E. phlebotomy
F. veins
G. antecubital space

Blood Collection—Capillary Puncture Terms

_____ 8. All the fluid except blood found in the space between tissues; also referred to as tissue fluid

_____ 9. A newborn child

_____ 10. Inflammation of the bone caused by bacterial infection

_____ 11. Abnormal collection of fluid in interstitial spaces

_____ 12. EDTA

_____ 13. A natural or synthesized chemical that prevents blood from clotting

_____ 14. Skin puncture or "stick" (typically finger stick on adults and heel stick on infants)

_____ 15. Process by which blood flows freely into a capillary tube in microcollection procedures

_____ 16. Condition in which the skin and mucous membranes are blue; caused by an oxygen deficiency

_____ 17. Lancet

_____ 18. A natural anticoagulant that prevents the blood from clotting

_____ 19. A test to detect bacteria or organisms growing in the blood

_____ 20. Collecting a small amount of blood

H. capillary action
I. osteomyelitis
J. microcollection
K. interstitial fluid
L. capillary puncture device
M. anticoagulant
N. blood culture
O. neonate
P. heparin
Q. capillary puncture
R. edema
S. cyanotic
T. A synthesized anticoagulant that also preserves the blood cells

Blood Collection—Venipuncture Terms

_____ 21. Liquid part of whole blood

_____ 22. Removing air to produce a vacuum

_____ 23. Inner tubular space of a needle, vessel, or tube

_____ 24. Immediately

_____ 25. Serum separator tube

_____ 26. Condition in which blood concentration of large molecules such as proteins, cells, and coagulation factors increases

_____ 27. Narrow middle layer of white blood cells and platelets in a centrifuged whole blood specimen

_____ 28. Plasma separator tube

_____ 29. A band placed above the venipuncture site

_____ 30. Liquid part obtained when blood is clotted; lacks the clotting factors

_____ 31. Tubes with air removed to produce a vacuum

A. plasma
B. serum
C. buffy coat
D. evacuating
E. hemoconcentration
F. PST
G. stat
H. evacuated tubes
I. lumen
J. SST
K. tourniquet

Advanced Concepts Terms

_____ 32. Tumor or swelling of blood in the tissues (resulting in bruising during blood collection procedures)

_____ 33. Tiny purple or red skin spots caused by small amounts of blood under the skin; found in patients with coagulation problems; can lead to excessive bleeding during phlebotomy procedures

_____ 34. The breaking open of red blood cells and the release of hemogobin

_____ 35. Fainting

_____ 36. Removal of a breast

L. mastectomy
M. hematoma
N. syncope
O. petechiae
P. hemolysis

FUNDAMENTAL CONCEPTS

37. Explain the differences between arteries, arterioles, capillaries, venules, and veins.

_____

_____

_____

_____

38. Determine whether the following substances are higher in the capillary or venous blood.

a. Hemoglobin _____

b. Total protein _____

c. Potassium _____

d. Glucose _____

e. Calcium _____

39. Describe the difference in the "feel" between an artery and a vein.

_____

_____

40. Draw a diagram of the most common veins in the antecubital area used for phlebotomy.

41. List the seven items that must be on a laboratory requisition or the patient's electronic record.

    a. _____

    b. _____

    c. _____

    d. _____

    e. _____

    f. _____

    g. _____

42. What is the most critical error that a phlebotomist can make before collecting the specimen?

_____

_____

43. Describe the three-way match for patient identification.

_____

_____

44. Explain the proper way to determine a patient's name.

_____

_____

45. Describe and explain the correct positions of a patient when performing phlebotomy.

_____

_____

Chapter **4** **Blood Collection**

Capillary Puncture

46. Describe the composition of capillary blood.

_____

_____

_____

47. Label the capillary puncture supplies (See a – f in Procedure 4.1 Capillary Puncture).

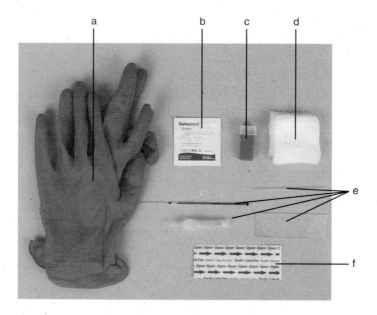

48. List three situations in which capillary blood may be used and three situations in which this method should not be used.

_____

_____

_____

_____

_____

_____

49. What is the recommended capillary puncture depth for newborns and infants? Explain why.

_____

_____

50. List the 6 types of point-of-care testing equipment that are used to collect the blood from capillary punctures. (Hint: See Figs. 4.6 in the textbook.)

_____

_____

51. List and explain the recommended order of collecting the various colored Microtainers from a capillary puncture. (Hint: See Table 4-2 in text)

_____

_____

_____

_____

52. Describe the appropriate capillary puncture collection sites for adults and children and for newborns and infants. (see Fig. 4.9 & Fig. 4.10 in textboook)

Adults and children: _____

_____

Infants and newborns: _____

_____

53. Why is the first drop of blood wiped away in a capillary puncture?

_____

_____

54. What are the effects of not allowing the alcohol to dry prior to performing the blood collection?

_____

_____

55. What will squeezing the puncture site do to the test results?

_____

_____

56. Describe what to do if the blood stops flowing and not enough blood was obtained.

_____

_____

57. Describe phenylketonuria (PKU).

_____

_____

58. Describe the neonatal screening collection procedure.

_____

_____

_____

_____

59. Discuss the infant age parameters for testing for PKU.

_____

_____

60. In the following case study steps, write **C** if the technique is correct or **I** if the technique is incorrect; explain why in the space provided.

A medical assistant performs a capillary puncture on an adult.

_____ 1. The medical assistant washes his or her hands and puts on gloves.

_____

_____ 2. The site that is chosen is the lateral part of the fingertip (slightly to the side of center) of the middle finger.

_____

_____ 3. The site is cleaned with 30% alcohol.

_____

_____ 4. The puncture is made before the site is dry.

_____

_____ 5. The puncture is made parallel to the whorls of the fingerprint.

_____

61. In the following scenario about a capillary puncture, circle the incorrect techniques. In the space provided, explain the repercussions that could occur from using the incorrect method.

A capillary puncture is performed on the central area of the heel of a newborn infant's foot. The area is cleaned with 70% alcohol; before the alcohol has dried, a puncture is made with a lancet to a depth of 3 mm. Immediately after the puncture, the blood is collected in a capillary tube by squeezing the puncture site. After all the blood has been obtained, pressure is applied to the puncture site, and an adhesive bandage is applied.

_____

_____

_____

_____

_____

62. Explain the difference between serum and plasma, and describe how each is obtained.

_____

_____

63. Label the parts of the Vacutainer system.

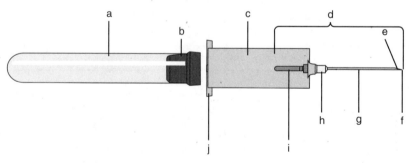

64. Place the following tubes in the correct order of draw and name the anticoagulant or additive in each: green, gray, red, lavender.

   a. _____; _____

   b. _____; _____

   c. _____; _____

   d. _____; _____

65. Describe how a gel separator tube functions for separating serum and for separating plasma from the cells.

   _____

   _____

66. Describe the function of the tourniquet. Include the appropriate distance from the puncture site a tourniquet should be placed and the recommended time it should be on the arm.

   _____

   _____

67. Discuss the criteria for determining whether a tourniquet has been placed correctly.

   _____

   _____

68. List the assets and limitations of the topical anesthetic EMLA.

   _____

   _____

69. Why should the tourniquet be released before removing the needle?

   _____

   _____

70. Why does the needle need to be held steady during a venipuncture procedure?

   _____

   _____

71. Name the three methods that can be used to obtain blood from a vein.

   _____

   _____

   _____

72. What are the most frequently used needle lengths and gauges for the Vacutainer system? Which gauge has a larger lumen, 21 or 23?

   _____

   _____

73. List the advantages of using the Vacutainer method.

_____

_____

74. Explain when a butterfly and syringe method would be used.

_____

_____

75. Describe the safety steps of discarding the needle after removing it from the arm with the Vacutainer method.

_____

_____

76. List three conditions that could cause a hematoma.

_____

_____

_____

77. Describe the recommended procedure for transferring blood from a syringe into vacuum tubes.

_____

_____

78. Describe the procedure for determining the appropriate vein for venipuncture.

_____

_____

79. Identify and describe the function of each part of the syringe system.

_____

_____

80. Label the parts of the syringe.

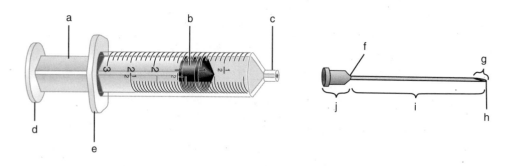

81. Identify and describe the function of each of the components of the butterfly system, including use of the Luer adapter/Vacutainer method and the syringe method.

_____

_____

82. Identify two quality assurance steps related to vacuum tube selection. (HINT: See Vacutainer Procedure 4.3 Preparation—Pre-analytical text.)

_____

_____

83. Discuss the Needle Stick Safety and Prevention Act passed by Congress, which directed the Occupational Safety and Health Administration (OSHA) to revise the bloodborne pathogens standards to require employers to identify and use safer medical devices.

_____

_____

84. In the following case study steps, write **C** if the technique is correct or **I** if the technique is incorrect, and explain why in the space provided.
    A medical assistant is performing a Vacutainer blood collection method.

    _____ 1. The patient is told to sit on the end of the examination table.

    _____

    _____ 2. The medical assistant washes his or her hands, puts on gloves, and then pops the top off of the index finger of the glove.

    _____

    _____ 3. The tourniquet is applied, and the median cubital vein is determined for use; the tourniquet is then removed.

    _____

    _____ 4. The chosen site is cleaned with 70% alcohol, working in concentric circles from the inside out, making sure not to backtrack. The tourniquet is then reapplied.

    _____

    _____ 5. The nondominant hand anchors the vein.

    _____

    _____ 6. The angle of the needle is 45 degrees as it enters the vein.

    _____

    _____ 7. After the needle is removed, the safety device is immediately activated.

    _____

    _____ 8. The needle is unscrewed from the holder and discarded in a sharps container, reusing the holder.

    _____

85. In the following scenario about a venipuncture procedure, circle the incorrect techniques. In the space provided, explain the seven repercussions that could occur from using the incorrect method.

A medical assistant examines an arm to determine the correct vein to use to obtain blood. The arm has very small veins. The medical assistant decides to use the Vacutainer method. The patient's name is determined by asking, "Are you Mrs. Jones?" The patient is then told to sit in a chair with an arm. All the tubes that will be drawn on this patient are prelabeled before the draw. After putting on the tourniquet approximately 3 inches above the puncture site, the arm is cleaned with 70% isopropyl alcohol, starting at the puncture site and moving in a concentric circles outward. The site is retouched by the phlebotomist without cleaning the finger. The needle is inserted into the vein at a 15-degree angle. The lavender tube is filled first, followed by the red tube and gray tube; the green tube is filled last. After the last tube is filled, the needle is removed from the vein, and the tourniquet is removed. Tubes are mixed approximately three times and placed in an upright position in the tray to be taken quickly to the laboratory to perform analytical testing.

_____

_____

_____

_____

_____

_____

_____

86. Label all the venipuncture supplies in the figure (see Fig. 4.23 in the textbook).

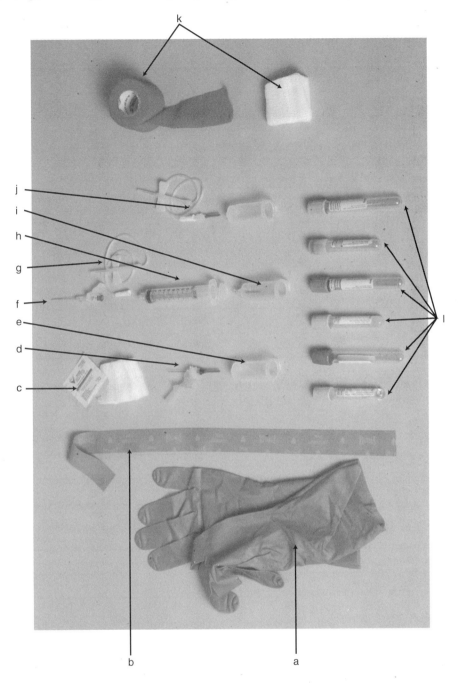

87. Internet activity: Visit one of the following Web sites and present your findings to the class.
www.mchb.hrsa.gov (Maternal and Child Health Bureau of the Health Resources and Services Administration)
www.aap.org (American Academy of Pediatrics)
www.bd.com (Becton Dickinson)
www.clsi.org
www.osha.gov (Occupational Safety and Health Administration)

88. The medical assistant is performing a Vacutainer procedure. The needle is inserted into the vein, and the vacuum tube is pushed into the Vacutainer holder. No blood is obtained. Discuss the five possible reasons why this occurred.

_____

_____

_____

89. During a venipuncture procedure, the patient becomes pale, sweats, and hyperventilates. Discuss what occurred and what should be done.

_____

_____

_____

90. The plasma in the vacuum tube appears pink. Explain what this is, list three things that can cause it, and name three tests that can be affected by this condition.

_____

_____

_____

91. After a needle was inserted into a patient's vein, the patient experienced a tingling sensation radiating down the arm. What occurred, and what should the phlebotomist do?

_____

_____

_____

92. If a patient has had a mastectomy, or has a broken arm, or has had an intravenous therapy in the arm on the left side of their body, why would you not draw blood from the left arm in each case?

Mastectomy: _____

Broken arm: _____

Intravenous therapy in the hand or lower arm: _____

93. List five ways to help successfully locate a vein in an obese person.

_____

_____

_____

_____

_____

BEHAVIORAL 4-1: Instructing Patients While Collecting Capillary Blood, or a Heel Stick Neonatal Screening Specimen, or a Vacutainer Blood Specimen, or a Syringe Method of Blood Collection, or a Butterfly Method of Collecting Blood.

Work in groups of four students each. Each student will play all the different roles in the blood-collecting procedures listed above. When acting as the medical assistant performing the procedure, sign the top line below and have three other students sign in with their respective roles (patient or evaluator). Each student should have at least one fully signed BEHAVIORAL evaluation turned in with one of the blood collection procedures in this chapter.

1. Medical assisting student being evaluated_____

2. Student playing the role of the patient_____

3. Student evaluator of Behavior: _____ (check Behavioral Procedure on the reverse side of this sheet based on your observations)

4. Student evaluator of Procedural steps: _____ (check off the Procedural section)

(Each evaluator needs to sign and date the forms)

COMPETENCY:	I.A.3. Show awareness of a patient's concerns related to procedure: _____ _____				
OBJECTIVE(s):	Given the conditions, and provided the necessary supplies, the student will demonstrate awareness of patient concerns as they provide patient care in a role-play scenario for a student-partner.				
TIME FRAME:	15 minutes				
GRADING:	**PASS = 100% accuracy.** All steps must be completed as written for "**PASS.**" Students are permitted two (2) graded attempts. **Grading Instructions:** When step is performed as written, record a "✓" for "**PASS.**" When step is omitted and/or there is an error in written procedure, record instructor initials for "**FAIL.**" Procedure must be repeated.				
		GRADED ATTEMPT 1		GRADED ATTEMPT 2	
STEP #	PROCEDURE (check the procedure you performed as a medical assistant student)	PASS	FAIL	PASS	FAIL
	___ 1. Capillary blood or heel stick collecion				
	___ 2. Vacutainer collection of blood				
	___ 3. Syringe collection of blood				
	___ 4. Butterfly collection of blood				
Example	Instructions to evaluator: Student **completes step** as written, record "✓" Student **omits step or performs it in error,** record initials	✓	ZH		
1.	Gathered supplies and reviewed the new or established patient's medical history form.				
2.	Correctly prepared the patient: ■ Greeted the patient, introduced self, escorted him/her to exam room, and verified name. ■ Made appropriate eye contact with the patient ■ Established a professional and empathetic atmosphere ■ Explained procedure to patient				
3.	Responded to patient concerns: ■ Showed empathy toward patient ■ Assured patient concerns are understood by repeating them and verifying them with patient ■ Explained procedure again to ensure patient understanding ■ Answered any questions from patient ■ Assured patient that procedure is necessary ■ Provided necessary follow-up contact information				

Evaluator signature _____   Procedure observed (1 – 4 above) _____

MA student signature _____   Date _____

Procedure 4.1: Capillary Puncture Procedure

Person evaluated _____ Date _____

Evaluated by _____

Outcome goal	To perform a capillary skin puncture with a retractable, nonreusable lancet
Conditions	Given the following supplies: - Sterile, disposable, retractable, nonreusable lancets (various lengths for the appropriate depth) - Microcollection containers, plastic capillary tubes (with anticoagulant), and sealers - Sterile gauze and 70% isopropyl alcohol pads in sterile packages - Gloves (latex and nonlatex for patients who are allergic) - Biohazard puncture-resistant sharps container - Warming devices, marking pen - Appropriate microcollection containers or testing devices or both depending on what test is ordered
Standards	Required time: 10 minutes Performance time: _____ Total possible points = _____ Points earned = _____
Evaluation Rubric Codes: **S** = Satisfactory, meets standard **U** = Unsatisfactory, fails to meet standard	
NOTE: Steps marked with an asterisk (*) are critical to achieve required competency.	

Preparation	Scores	
	S	**U**
*1. Identified patient and placed in proper position.		
- Had patient state name.		
- Confirmed identification with patient (birth date or picture ID).		
- Compared with requisition.		
2. Sanitized hands and put on gloves.		
3. Determined the most suitable puncture site and warmed the site.		
- A finger stick: third and fourth finger should be used, making the puncture on the lateral part of the fingertip (slightly to the side of center) and perpendicular to the fingerprint.		
- Newborn or infant (not walking): the medial or lateral plantar section of the foot should be used.		
- Warmed area by massaging the areas five or six times or applied a warmed towel, preemie diaper, or a commercially available device to the site for 3 to 5 minutes.		

Procedure	Scores	
	S	**U**
*4. Disinfected area over chosen site and assembled equipment.		
- Cleaned the site with 70% alcohol.		
- Allowed to dry without fanning or blowing on cleansed site.		
- Assembled the capillary equipment needed, determining the appropriate lancet device to use according to the age and amount of blood needed.		
- Placed all supplies in close proximity to hand.		

5. Pressing hard, made a puncture in the cleaned area at the appropriate site.		
*6. Wiped away the first drop of blood.		
*7. Collected the blood in the proper container by the correct technique.		
- Collected free-flowing drops of blood; did not scoop, scrape, or squeeze the site.		
- If blood was collected in a capillary tube, held the tube horizontal to the site and did not have any air bubbles.		

	Scores	
Follow-up	S	U
8. Asked the patient to apply pressure to site for 3 to 5 minutes.		
9. Gently mixed microcontainers by tilting 8 to 10 times, and labeled all tubes properly.		
- Marked date and time of draw, patient name, and initials or name of phlebotomist.		
- Placed capillary tubes in a vacuum tube, and labeled the vacuum tube.		
10. Checked site for bleeding, and applied pressure bandage to site.		
- If bleeding continued after 5 minutes, contacted physician.		
- Checked if patient was allergic to bandages before application.		
- Informed parent, if patient is a child, to remove the adhesive bandage after bleeding has stopped, because children may choke on it if it is placed in the mouth.		
11. Determined whether patient was feeling well before dismissing.		
*12. Completed proper documentation on patient chart (see below).		
13. Properly performed disposal and disinfection.		
- Disposed of all sharps in biohazard sharps containers.		
- Disposed of regulated medical waste in biohazard bags (gloves, gauze).		
- Disinfected test area and instruments according to OSHA guidelines.		
14. Sanitized hands.		
Total Points per Column		

Patient Name: _____

Patient Chart Entry: (Include when, what, how, why, any additional information, and the signature of the person charting. See example in the textbook.)

_____

_____

_____

Procedure 4.2: Heel Stick for Neonatal Screening Test Procedure

Person evaluated _____ Date _____

Evaluated by _____

Outcome goal	Perform a capillary skin puncture with a retractable, nonreusable lancet
Conditions	Given the following supplies: - Gloves (preferably nonlatex for latex-sensitive patients) - Sterile gauze - Warming device - 70% isopropyl alcohol pads in sterile packages - Sterile, disposable, retractable, nonreusable neonatal lancets with no more than 2-mm depth - Neonatal screening filter paper
Standards	Required time: 15 minutes Performance time: _____ Total possible points = _____ Points earned = _____

Evaluation Rubric Codes:
S = Satisfactory, meets standard   **U** = Unsatisfactory, fails to meet standard

NOTE: Steps marked with an asterisk (*) are critical to achieve required competency.

Preparation	Scores S	Scores U
*1. Washed the hands if they were visibly soiled. If not, used an alcohol-based rub for routine decontamination. Applied the hand rub to the palm of one hand and rubbed the hands together, covering all surfaces until dry.		
*2. Correctly identified the newborn by using the three-way match, and filled out all the information required on the card.		
*3. Applied gloves.		
*4. Chose the appropriate site for the heel stick according to the guidelines.		
- Newborn or infant (not walking): the medial or lateral plantar section of the foot should be used.		
- Applied a warmed towel, preemie diaper, or a commercially available device to the site for 3 to 5 minutes.		

Procedure	Scores S	Scores U
*5. Cleaned the site with 70% isopropyl alcohol. Allowed the alcohol to dry, without fanning or blowing on the site.		
*6. With a gloved hand, placed the lancet against the medial or lateral plantar surface of the heel of the foot.		
*7. Placed the blade slot area securely against the heel, and firmly and completely depressed the lancet trigger.		
*8. Gently wiped away the first drop of blood with sterile gauze or cotton ball.		
*9. Applied gentle pressure with the thumb and eased pressure intermittently as drops of blood formed. Applied pressure in such a way that the incision site remained open.		

Chapter **4 Blood Collection**

		Scores
		S	U
*10. The filter paper should be touched gently against the large blood drop, and in one step, a sufficient quantity of blood should soak through to fill a preprinted circle on the filter paper completely.			
- Do not reapply additional drops in the same circle after leaving the circle.			
- The paper should not be pressed or smeared against the puncture site of the heel.			
- Blood should be applied only to one side of the filter paper, but both sides of the filter paper should be examined to ensure that the blood uniformly saturated the paper.			
*11. After all five circles of blood have been collected from the heel of the newborn, the foot should be elevated above the body.			
NOTE: A minimum of three successful circles is needed by the laboratory to test for multiple metabolic disorders.			
*12. A sterile gauze pad or cotton swab should be pressed against the puncture site until the bleeding stops.			
- It is not advisable to apply adhesive bandages over skin puncture sites on newborns.			

Follow-up	Scores	
	S	U
*13. Logged and charted the procedure.		
*14. Allowed filter paper to dry thoroughly on a horizontal, level, nonabsorbent open surface for 3 hours at ambient temperature and away from direct sunlight.		
- Do not touch or smear blood on the filter paper, and do not contaminate the specimen card with cleaning chemicals or other substances.		
- Mailed the thoroughly dried card (Fig. F in textbook, Procedure 4.2) in the envelope provided by the health department.		
- Placed capillary tubes in a vacuum tube and labeled the vacuum tube.		
*15. Properly performed disposal and disinfection.		
- Disposed of all sharps in biohazard sharps containers.		
- Disposed of regulated medical waste in biohazard bags (gloves, gauze).		
- Disinfected test area and instruments according to OSHA guidelines.		
16. Sanitized hands.		
Total Points per Column		

Patient Name: _____

Patient Chart Entry: (Include when, what, how, why, any additional information, and the signature of the person charting.)

_____

_____

_____

Procedure 4.3: Vacutainer Method

Person evaluated _____ Date _____

Evaluated by _____

Outcome goal	Perform a venipuncture by the Vacutainer method
Conditions	Given the following supplies: - Disposable gloves - Tourniquet - 70% isopropyl alcohol and sterile gauze pads - Vacutainer double-pointed needle and Vacutainer holder - Correct vacuum tubes for requested tests - Adhesive bandages - Test tube rack - Biohazard sharps containers and bags
Standards	Required time: 10 minutes Performance time: _____ Total possible points = _____ Points earned = _____

Evaluation Rubric Codes:
S = Satisfactory, meets standard   **U** = Unsatisfactory, fails to meet standard

NOTE: Steps marked with an asterisk (*) are critical to achieve required competency.

Preparation	Scores	
	S	**U**
*1. Identified and placed patient in proper position.		
- Had patient state name.		
- Confirmed identification with patient (birth date or picture ID).		
- Compared identification with requisition.		
2. Sanitized hands and put on gloves.		
3. Applied tourniquet and determined the most suitable puncture site.		
- Used sufficient pressure to stop venous flow but not arterial flow.		
- Palpated and determined size, depth, and direction of vein.		
4. Removed tourniquet, disinfected area over chosen site, and assembled equipment.		
- Cleansed the site with 70% isopropyl alcohol in concentric circles from inside out.		
- Allowed alcohol to dry without fanning or blowing on cleansed site.		
- Connected the venipuncture assembly in a sterile manner.		
- Placed all supplies in close proximity to arm.		

Procedure	Scores	
	S	**U**
5. Reapplied tourniquet and instructed patient to make a fist (no pumping).		
*6. Disinfected gloved fingers if necessary to palpate site again.		
*7. Uncovered needle, anchored vein, and inserted needle.		
- Pulled skin taut with nondominant thumb 1 to 2 inches below and to the side of the puncture site.		
- Inserted needle ¼ to ½ inch below the vein with bevel up in one swift, continuous motion with dominant hand.		

Chapter **4** **Blood Collection**

	S	U
*8. Pushed tube into needle holder.		
- Used the index and middle fingers of nondominant hand on both sides of the flange and pushed the tube with the thumb of the same hand.		
*9. Followed proper order of draw when filling, removing, and mixing the tubes.		
- Used thumb of nondominant hand against flange and pulled tube out with the fingers of the same hand.		
- Inverted each tube gently to mix blood with additives.		
- Removed the last tube to prevent blood dripping from needle.		
- Instructed patient to release fist.		
*10. Removed tourniquet before taking needle out of arm.		
*11. Placed sterile gauze over needle as it was pulled out and then applied pressure to site.		
- Did not press on gauze until after needle was removed.		
*12. Immediately activated needle safety device and discarded Vacutainer and needle as a unit into the sharps container.		

Follow-up	Scores	
	S	U
13. Asked the patient to apply pressure to site for 3 to 5 minutes.		
14. Gently mixed tubes by tilting 8 to 10 times, and labeled all tubes properly.		
- Marked patient name, date and time of draw, and initials or name of phlebotomist.		
*15. Checked site for bleeding, and applied pressure bandage to site.		
- If bleeding continued after 5 minutes, contacted physician.		
- Checked if patient was allergic to bandages before application.		
16. Determined if patient was feeling well before dismissing.		
17. Completed proper documentation on patient chart (see below).		
*18. Properly disposed of or disinfected materials.		
- Disposed of all sharps in biohazard sharp containers.		
- Disposed of regulated medical waste (e.g., gloves, gauze) in biohazard bags.		
- Disinfected of test area and instruments according to OSHA guidelines.		
19. Sanitized hands.		
Total Points per Column		

Patient Name: _____

Patient Chart Entry: (Include when, what, how, why, any additional information, and the signature of the person charting.)

_____

_____

_____

Procedure 4.4: Syringe Method

Person evaluated _____ Date _____

Evaluated by _____

Outcome goal	Perform a venipuncture by the syringe method
Conditions	Given the following supplies: - Disposable gloves - Tourniquet - 70% isopropyl alcohol and sterile gauze pads - Proper-size syringe and needle - Safety transfer device - Correct vacuum tubes for requested tests - Adhesive bandages - Test tube rack - Biohazard sharps containers and bags
Standards	Required time: 10 minutes Performance time: _____ Total possible points = _____ Points earned = _____

Evaluation Rubric Codes:
S = Satisfactory, meets standard   **U** = Unsatisfactory, fails to meet standard

NOTE: Steps marked with an asterisk (*) are critical to achieve required competency.

Preparation	Scores	
	S	**U**
*1. Identified and placed patient in proper position.		
- Had patient state name.		
- Confirmed identification with patient (birth date or picture ID).		
- Compared identification with requisition.		
2. Sanitized hands and put on gloves.		
3. Applied tourniquet and determined the most suitable puncture site.		
- Applied sufficient pressure to stop venous flow but not arterial flow.		
- Palpated and determined size, depth, and direction of vein.		
4. Removed tourniquet, disinfected area over chosen site, and assembled equipment.		
- Cleansed site with 70% isopropyl alcohol in concentric circles from inside out.		
- Allowed alcohol to dry without fanning or blowing on cleansed site.		
- Connected the syringe assembly in a sterile manner.		
- Placed all supplies in close proximity to arm.		

Procedure	Scores	
	S	**U**
*5. Reapplied tourniquet and instructed patient to make a fist (no pumping).		
- Disinfected gloved fingers if necessary to palpate site again.		

	Scores	
	S	U
*6. Removed needle cover, anchored vein, and inserted needle.		
- Pulled skin taut with nondominant thumb 1 to 2 inches below and to the side of the puncture site.		
- Inserted needle ¼ to ½ inch below the vein with bevel up in one swift, continuous motion with dominant hand at the appropriate angle.		
*7. Gently pulled syringe plunger back.		
- Was careful not to pull out of the vein.		
- Instructed patient to release fist.		
*8. Removed tourniquet before taking needle out of arm.		
*9. Placed sterile gauze over needle as it was pulled out, then applied pressure to site.		
- Did not press on the gauze until after the needle was removed.		
*10. Immediately activated syringe needle safety device, unscrewed the needle, and discarded it into the sharps container.		

	Scores	
Follow-up	S	U
11. Asked the patient to apply pressure with gauze to site for 3 to 5 minutes.		
12. Filled the vacuum tubes in the proper order of draw by using a transfer safety device.		
- Did not push on the plunger.		
13. Gently mixed tubes by tilting 8 to 10 times, and labeled all tubes properly.		
- Marked patient name, date and time of draw, and initials or name of phlebotomist.		
*14. Checked site for bleeding and applied pressure bandage to site.		
- If bleeding continued after 5 minutes, contacted physician.		
- Checked if patient was allergic to bandages before application.		
15. Determined if patient was feeling well before dismissing.		
16. Completed proper documentation on patient chart (see below).		
*17. Properly disposed of or disinfected materials.		
- Disposed of all sharps, including the transfer device or syringe, in biohazard sharps container.		
- Disposed of regulated medical waste in biohazard bags (gloves, gauze).		
- Disinfected test area and instruments according to OSHA guidelines.		
18. Sanitized hands.		
Total Points per Column		

Patient Name: _____

Patient Chart Entry: (Don't forget to include when, how, what, why, any additional information, and the signature of the person charting.)

_____

_____

_____

Procedure 4.5: Two Butterfly Methods From a Hand and Training Model

Person evaluated _____ Date _____

Evaluated by _____

Outcome goal	Perform a venipuncture by the butterfly method
Conditions	Given the following supplies: - Disposable gloves, tourniquet, 70% isopropyl alcohol, and gauze pads - Winged butterfly set (Safety-Lock or Push Button) with syringe adapter and Vacutainer adapter - Proper-size syringe or Vacutainer holder - Correct vacuum tubes for requested tests - Adhesive bandages - Test tube rack and biohazard sharps containers and bags
Standards	Required time: 10 minutes Performance time: _____ Total possible points = _____ Points earned = _____
Evaluation Rubric Codes: **S** = Satisfactory, meets standard **U** = Unsatisfactory, fails to meet standard	
NOTE: Steps marked with an asterisk (*) are critical to achieve required competency.	

Preparation	Scores S	Scores U
*1. Identified and placed patient in proper position.		
- Had patient state name.		
- Confirmed identification with patient (birth date or picture ID).		
- Compared identification with requisition.		
2. Sanitized hands and put on gloves.		
3. Applied tourniquet and determined the most suitable puncture site.		
- Applied sufficient pressure to stop venous flow but not arterial flow.		
- Palpated and determined size, depth, and direction of vein.		
4. Removed tourniquet, disinfected area over chosen site, and assembled equipment.		
- Cleansed site with 70% isopropyl alcohol in concentric circles from inside out.		
- Allowed alcohol to dry without fanning or blowing on cleansed site.		
- Straightened out the butterfly tubing.		
- Connected the venipuncture butterfly assembly in a sterile manner to a syringe or a Vacutainer holder.		
- Pushed the plunger back and forth to break the seal if attaching a syringe.		
- Placed all supplies in close proximity to arm or hand.		

Procedure	Scores S	Scores U
*5. Reapplied the tourniquet and disinfected gloved fingers if necessary to palpate site again.		
*6. Removed needle sheath, anchored vein, and inserted needle.		
- Pulled skin taut with nondominant thumb 1 to 2 inches below and to the side of the puncture site.		
- Held the butterfly wings together with the dominant hand and inserted needle ¼ to ½ inch below the vein with bevel up in one swift, continuous motion with dominant hand at the appropriate angle.		

85

	S	U
*7. Used the correct technique to obtain blood.		
- Gently pulled syringe plunger back if using syringe method.		
- Used the index and middle fingers of nondominant hand on both sides of the flange and pushed the tube into the holder with the thumb of the same hand if the Vacutainer method was used.		
*8. Tourniquet removed before taking needle out of arm.		
*9. Placed sterile gauze over needle as it was pulled out and then applied pressure to site.		
- Did not press on the gauze until after the needle was removed.		
*10. Immediately activated butterfly needle safety device in a safe manner and disposed of butterfly apparatus properly (illustrations show how to activate the Safety Lock and the Push Button safety devices).		
- If Vacutainer method was used, the butterfly needle, tubing, and Vacutainer holder were discarded in a biohazard sharps container.		
- If a syringe method was used, the syringe was removed from the butterfly tubing, and the butterfly needle and tubing were discarded into a biohazard sharps container.		

Follow-up	Scores	
	S	U
11. Asked the patient to apply pressure with gauze to site for 3 to 5 minutes.		
12. Filled the vacuum tubes in the proper order of draw by using a transfer safety device if syringe method was used.		
- Did not push on plunger; let vacuum fill the tube.		
13. Gently mixed tubes by tilting 8 to 10 times, and labeled all tubes properly.		
- Marked patient name, date and time of draw, and initials or name of phlebotomist.		
*14. Checked site for bleeding and applied pressure bandage to site.		
- If bleeding continued after 5 minutes, contacted physician.		
- Checked if patient was allergic to bandages before application.		
15. Determined if patient was feeling well before dismissing.		
16. Completed proper documentation on patient chart (see below).		
*17. Properly disposed of or disinfected equipment.	*18.	*19.
- Disposed of all sharps, including the transfer device and syringe (if syringe method was used), in biohazard sharps containers.		
- Disposed of regulated medical waste (e.g., gloves, gauze) in biohazard bags.		
- Disinfected test area and instruments according to OSHA guidelines.		
18. Sanitized hands.		
Total Points per Column		

Patient Name: _____

Patient Chart Entry: (Include when, what, how, why, any additional information, and the signature of the person charting.)

_____

_____

Procedure 4.6: Possible Final Practical Exam for this Chapter.

COMPETENCY:	I.A.3. Show awareness of a patient's concerns related to the procedure being performed V.A.4. Explain to a patient the rationale for performing the venipuncture and/or capillary puncture I.A.2. Incorporate critical thinking skills and documentation skills when performing venipuncture and capillary puncture
OBJECTIVE(s):	Given the conditions, and provided the necessary phlebotomy supplies, the student will demonstrate awareness of patient concerns, explain the rationale for performing venipuncture and capillary puncture, and incorporate critical thinking skills as they provide patient care in a role-play scenario with a student-partner.
SUPPLIES:	Predetermined patient scenarios (patient presents to office for a visit and to have their blood drawn via capillary puncture or venipuncture). The instructor will provide: a simulated patient chart (electronic or paper) and lab order for a test needing a blood sample. NOTE: The following scenarios are for developing patient rapport; therefore, simulated models may be used during the following interactive scenarios: 1. A scared child needing a finger stick for glucose test 2. An infant needing a heel stick for newborn screening 3. A nauseated pregnant woman needing blood drawn and sent to the lab for hematology and chemistry testing 5. An outspoken man who says he always faints at the sight of blood needs a venipuncture for coagulation testing 4. An elderly patient who is confused and needs a venipuncture from the hand using a butterfly needle and syringe for a chemistry profile 6. A non-English-speaking patient who is very frail and whose veins are difficult to see has a helper who says she always has her blood drawn with a butterfly needle
TIME FRAME:	15 minutes
GRADING:	**PASS = 100% accuracy;** All steps must be completed as written for "**PASS.**" Students are permitted two (2) graded attempts. **Grading Instructions:** When step is performed as written, record a "✓" for "**PASS.**" When step is omitted and/or there is an error in written product, record instructor initials for "**FAIL.**" Procedure must be repeated.
WORK PRODUCT:	The appropriate Vacutainer tubes for the tests ordered, labeled correctly, and packaged for the lab to pick up. Documentation in patient's record and on the lab log.
PRECAUTIONS:	To act in accordance with OSHA regulations, appropriate Standard Precautions must be observed when there is the possibility of contact with blood or bodily fluids.

		GRADED ATTEMPT 1		GRADED ATTEMPT 2	
STEP #	**PROCEDURE: Interacting with**	PASS	FAIL	PASS	FAIL
Ex.	Student **completes step** as written, record "✓"in PASS column Student **omits step or performs it in error,** record initials in FAIL column				
1.	Gathered supplies and reviewed the new or established patient's medical history form.				
2.	Correctly prepared the patient: ■ Greeted the patient, introduced self, escorted him/her to exam room, and verified name. ■ Made appropriate eye contact with the patient ■ Established a professional and empathetic atmosphere ■ Explained procedure to patient				

87

3.	Responded to patient concerns: ■ Showed empathy toward patient ■ Assured that they understood concerns by repeating them and verifying them with patient ■ Answered any questions from patient ■ Assured patient that procedure is necessary				
4.	Performed the procedure ■ Communicated with patient appropriately and with ease throughout task ■ Incorporated critical thinking skills ■ Groomed appearance and appropriate attire ■ Used the appropriate Vacutainer tubes for the tests ordered, labeled them correctly, and packaged them for the lab to pick up. ■ Proper documentation in patient's record and on the lab log				

Vacuum Tube Exercise

Visualize the following picture:

- *Blue* sky is at the top and is the first tube to draw.
- The *red and gold* rays of the sun are on the horizon. They both must be drawn *after* the blue but *before* the remaining anticoagulant tubes.
- *Green* grassy hill is located below the sun rays.
- *Lavender* flowers are at the bottom of the hill growing above the rocks.
- *Gray* rocks are at the bottom of the picture because gray is the last tube to draw.

Next, fill in the blank boxes and missing words from Table 4-5 in the textbook. Cut the rows, mix them up, and then place back in order, or cut all the boxes and put them back together like a puzzle.

Colors in Mountain Picture Placed in Order of Draw from Top to Bottom	Tube Descriptions	Additives	Laboratory Uses
_____ sky at the top	"_____" = tube		_____
_____ and _____ rays above the mountain	red topped tubes = "_____" tube	clot activator in plastic tubes (red *glass* tubes do not have clot activator)	both yield serum commonly used for testing blood
	gold topped (or red/gray) = "_____" tube	_____ and	
	light green topped (or green/gray) "_____" tube	with lithium or sodium (and gel in the PST tubes)	special tests such as _____
_____ grass on the mountain	dark green "_____" tube		
_____ flowers at the base of the mountain	"_____" tube		
_____ rocks at the bottom	"_____" tube		_____ testing

5 Hematology

VOCABULARY REVIEW

Match each definition with the correct term located on this page.

_____	1. Large nuclear cell in the bone marrow that fragments its cytoplasm to become platelets	A. anisocytosis
_____	2. Stem cell in the bone marrow that develops into the three kinds of granulocytes	B. baso-
_____	3. Abnormally shaped	C. differentiate
_____	4. Prefix meaning acid	D. eosino-
_____	5. Prefix meaning alkaline (base)	E. erythroblasts
_____	6. Also called rubriblasts, which become red blood cells	F. formed elements
_____	7. Suffix meaning attraction	G. granulocytes
_____	8. Blood production	H. hematologists
_____	9. Cells and cell fragments that can be viewed under the microscope	I. hematopoiesis
_____	10. Specialists who evaluate the cellular elements of blood microscopically and analytically	J. hemocytoblast
_____	11. Large, engulfing cells in the tissues that come from monocytes	K. macrophages
_____	12. Many-shaped nucleus; also called PMN or seg	L. myeloblast
_____	13. White blood cell group: Neutrophils, basophils, and eosinophils group	M. nuclei
_____	14. Newly released red blood cells in the blood that still contain some nuclear DNA	N. -phil
_____	15. Stem cell capable of becoming any of the blood cells	O. poikilocytosis
_____	16. To change and become something different	P. polymorphonuclear
_____	17. Variances in red blood cell size	Q. reticulocytes
_____	18. Platelets	R. thrombocytes
_____	19. Lymphocytes and monocytes group	S. megakaryocyte

NOTE: Additional definitions and their terms are continued on the next page

_____ 20. A critical element in the production of prothrombin

_____ 21. Fluid in the cell containing the nucleus and organells

_____ 22. Abnormal condition of increased red blood cells

_____ 23. Abnormal decrease in white blood cells

_____ 24. Abnormal increase in white blood cells

_____ 25. Abnormal condition of internal clotting

_____ 26. Condition in which the red blood cell or hemoglobin levels are below normal

_____ 27. Destruction of the red blood cells

_____ 28. Lack of oxygen in the blood

_____ 29. RBCs grouping together like stacked chips

_____ 30. Mathematic ratios of the three red blood cell tests (hemoglobin, hematocrit, and red blood cell count)

_____ 31. Ability of blood to maintain the balance of initiating a clotting response to stop bleeding and at the same time prevent the blood from forming an unwanted stationary clot

_____ 32. Two plasma proteins involved in clotting

_____ 33. Percentage of the five kinds of white blood cells

_____ 34. Cancer of the white blood cells

_____ 35. Increase in color (based on hemoglobin concentration)

_____ 36. test for monitoring coagulation times for patients taking anticoagulants such as coumadin

A. anemia
B. cytoplasm
C. fibrinogen, prothrombin
D. hemolysis
E. hemostasis
F. hypoxemia
G. leukemia
H. leukocytosis
I. leukopenia
J. hyperchromic
K. RBC indices
L. protime test
M. rouleaux formation
N. thrombosis
O. vitamin K
P. differential count
Q. polycythemia

FUNDAMENTAL CONCEPTS

37. Blood collected from a(n) _____ or a(n) _____ may be used for routine hematologic procedures.

38. The anticoagulated Vacutainer tube containing _____ with a(n) _____ top is used for most hematology tests.

39. Match each blood component with its associated characteristic.

_____ basophil   A Able to engulf foreign matter, especially bacteria

_____ erythrocyte   B. Increases in number during allergic reactions

_____ monocyte   C. Can differentiate into a T cell or a B cell

_____ neutrophil   D. Enters the tissues to mediate the inflammatory response

_____ platelet   E. Gathers around the site of a damaged blood vessel and releases chemicals to stimulate clot formation

_____ lymphocyte   F. Carries oxygen from the lungs to the cells of the body

_____ eosinophil   G. Becomes a macrophage when it leaves the blood to clean up debris in the tissues

40. Label the missing elements of the following hematopoiesis chart (see Fig. 5.3 in the textbook).

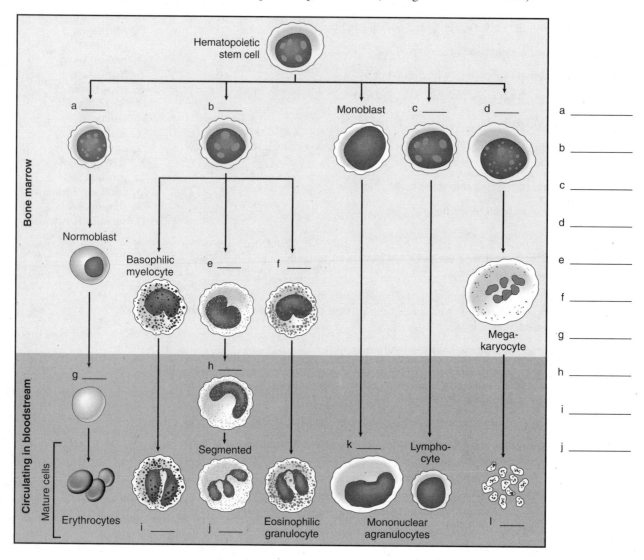

Preparation of a Blood Smear

41. A properly done blood smear will have a(n) _____ edge at the thin end of the slide and a section containing well-distributed blood cells in the _____ of the slide.

42. Blood smears are observed under the _____ lens.

43. When identifying cells, what three characteristics should the technician observe? (Hint: The *RBC Atlas* and *WBC Atlas* describe the general characteristics to observe in blood cells.)

_____

_____

Chapter **5** Hematology

Hemostasis

44. Explain the involvement of each of the following as they pertain to hemostasis. (Hint: See Fig. 5-9.)

Blood vessels: _____

Platelets: _____

Clotting factors: _____

Anticoagulants: _____

45. What is the difference between a thrombus and an embolus?

_____

_____

PROCEDURES: CLIA-WAIVED HEMATOLOGY TESTS

Hemoglobin

46. The two main components of hemoglobin are _____ and _____.

47. What is the function of hemoglobin? _____

Hematocrit

48. Match the following average hematocrit percentages to each population, and note the highest to the lowest averages.

_____ Normal average hematocrit for a woman   A. 56%

_____ Normal average hematocrit for a 6-year-old child   B. 42%

_____ Normal average hematocrit for a man   C. 38%

_____ Normal average hematocrit for a newborn   D. 47%

49. If a sample of capillary blood is used for the microhematocrit, the capillary tube must contain a(n) _____.

50. One medical condition in which a low hematocrit value may be found is _____.

51. True or false: Spun hematocrits should be performed in duplicate. _____

52. Label the layers of the spun hematocrit tube.

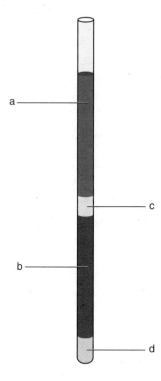

Erythrocyte Sedimentation Rate

53. What medical conditions can cause an increased erythrocyte sedimentation rate (ESR)?

_____

_____

54. What technical interferences during testing would cause an increased erythrocyte sedimentation rate?

_____

_____

Prothrombin Time

55. Describe the role of prothrombin in blood coagulation.

_____

_____

56. Explain the major use of the prothrombin time test.

_____

_____

57. Match each test with its reference range.

_____ hemoglobin   A. 36% to 55%

_____ hematocrit   B. 0 to 20 mm/hr

_____ ProTime   C. 12 to 18 g/dL

_____ ESR   D. Approximately 9 to 18 seconds, or 2 to 2.5 INR

58. Label the HemoCue equipment and supplies (see Procedure 5.2 -A in the textbook).

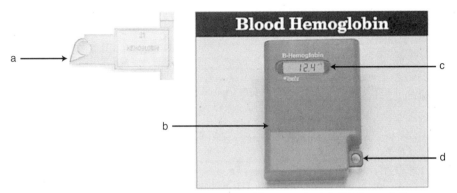

After approximately 15–45 seconds the result is displayed.

59. Label the SEDIPLAST ESR supplies (see Procedure 5.5-A in the textbook).

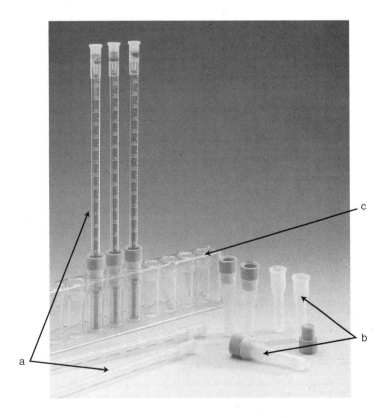

60. List the seven tests that comprise the complete blood count.

_____

_____

_____

_____

_____

_____

_____

61. What changes in blood cell size are caused by deficiency of vitamin B_{12}? (Hint: Look under "Anemias" in the textbook.)

_____

_____

62. List two conditions in which anisocytosis is found. (Hint: Look under "Anemias" in the textbook.)

_____

_____

63. Match the red blood cell indices to their reference ranges. (Hint: See Table 5.1, ADULTS column, and note the units associated with each test.)

_____ MCV   A. 26 to 34 pg

_____ MCH   B. 31% to 37% or g/dL

_____ MCHC   C. 82 to 98 μm or fL

64. Hypochromic, microcytic red blood cells have a (higher or lower) _____ MCV and (higher or lower) _____ MCHC.

65. Why does anemia or thrombocytopenia develop in patients with leukemia? (Hint: Consider where and how hematopoiesis occurs.)

_____

_____

66. Name one cause of eosinophilia. (Hint: Review granulocyte functions in "Fundamental Concepts.")

_____

_____

67. Name one cause of neutrophilia. (Hint: Review granulocyte functions in "Fundamental Concepts.")

_____

_____

68. Match the cell with its differential ADULT reference percentage according to Table 5.1 in your textbook, circle the two cells with the highest percentages, and underline the two cells with the lowest percentages.

_____ band   A. 3% to 9%

_____ lymphocyte   B. 50% to 65%

_____ neutrophil   C. 0% to 7%

_____ monocyte   D. 0% to 1%

_____ eosinophil   E. 25% to 40%

_____ basophil   F. 1% to 3%

Procedure 5.1: Diff Staining Procedure

Person evaluated _____ Date _____

Evaluated by _____

Outcome goal	Demonstrate the proper staining of a blood smear
Conditions	Given the following supplies: - smeared blood slide (see Figs. 5.10, 5.11, 5.12, and 5.13 in the textbook) - Quick Diff stain: fixative, red eosin dye, blue baso dye - staining rack - water source (bottled or running water) - bibulous paper - personal protective equipment—gown and gloves
Standards	Required time: 10 minutes Performance time: _____ Total possible points = _____ Points earned = _____
Evaluation Rubric Codes: **S** = Satisfactory, meets standard **U** = Unsatisfactory, fails to meet standard	
NOTE: Steps marked with an asterisk (*) are critical to achieve required competency.	

Preparation	Scores	
	S	**U**
1. Put on personal protective equipment (PPE).		

Procedure	Scores	
	S	**U**
2. Dip the slide in fixative three to five times and allow it to dry completely.		
3. Dip the slide into the red eosin dye three to five times.		
4. Let the excess dye run off and blot the rest away with absorbent paper.		
5. Dip the slide into the blue baso dye three to five times.		
6. After the blue dye is blotted away, rinse the slide thoroughly with water on both sides and allow it to air dry. It may also be pressed between two bibulous papers to help remove the water.		

Follow-up	Scores	
	S	**U**
*7. Observe the slide under the oil immersion lens of the microscope. The challenge is to find the WBCs.		
- Refer to the microscope skill sheet in Chapter 2 for the proper steps to bring the slide into focus under the oil immersion lens.		
- The cells and platelets will be enlarged 1000 times (100× oil objective times the 10 × ocular lens).		
- The slide will show predominantly RBCs with some small platelet clumps throughout.		
- The two most commonly found WBCs are segmented neutrophils and small lymphocytes.		
- See WHITE BLOOD CELL ATLAS for assistance in identifying the WBCs.		
Totals Counts per Column		

Patient Name: _____

Patient Chart Entry: (Include when, what, why, any additional information, and the signature of the person charting.)

_____

_____

_____

Procedure 5.2: Hemoglobin: HemoCue Method

Person evaluated _____ Date _____

Evaluated by _____

Outcome goal	To perform FDA-approved CLIA-waived Hemoglobin test following the most current OSHA safety guidelines and applying the correct quality control
Conditions	Given - HemoCue Instrument - Control cuvette - Microcuvette testing devices - Liquid controls: high and low - Alcohol, gauze, safety lancets, and bandage - Personal protective equipment
	Required time: 10 minutes Performance time: _____ Total possible points = _____ Points earned = _____
Evaluation Rubric Codes: **S** = Satisfactory, meets standard **U** = Unsatisfactory, fails to meet standard	
NOTE: Steps marked with an asterisk (*) are critical to achieve required competency.	

Preparation: Preanalytical Phase	Scores	
	S	U
A. Test information		
- Kit or instrument method: **HemoCue hemoglobin**		
- Manufacturer: **HemoCue**		
- Proper storage (e.g., temperature, light): **cuvettes stored at room temperature**		
- Lot number on cuvette container: _____		
- Expiration date: _____ **(opened container is stable for 3 months)**		
- Test flow chart _____ yes _____ no		
B. Specimen information		
- Type of specimen: **capillary blood or EDTA tube blood**		
- Testing device: **microcuvette test device**		
C. Personal protective equipment: **gloves, gown, sharps, and biohazard container or biohazard bag.**		
D. Assembled all equipment, sanitized hands, and applied personal protective equipment		

Procedure: Analytical Phase	Scores	
	S	U
E. Performed/observed quality control		
1. Quantitative testing controls (if testing method does not have internal controls)		
- Calibration check: **used control cuvette for optics check**		
- Results of Control levels: high _____ low _____		

F. Performed patient test		
1. Followed proper steps (from test flow chart).		
2. Obtained sufficient drop of blood properly.		
- Wiped away first drop and allowed new drop to form.		
3. Filled cuvette completely in one continuous process; did not top off.		
4. Wiped off excess blood on outside of cuvette immediately.		
- Avoided pulling out blood by contacting tip of cuvette while wiping away the excess blood.		
5. Visually inspected for air bubbles and loss of blood from cuvette.		
6. Placed filled cuvette into the cuvette holder and pushed holder into the measuring position.		
7. Result displayed after 30 to 60 seconds.		
***Accurate Results _____ Instructor Confirmation _____**		

Follow-up: Postanalytical Phase	Scores	
	S	**U**
***G. Proper documentation**		
1. On control log _____ yes _____ no		
2. On patient log _____ yes _____ no		
3. Documented on patient chart (see below)		
4. Identified critical values and took appropriate steps to notify physician - Hemoglobin expected values: Men = 13.0 to 18 g/dL Women = 11.0 to 16.0 g/dL Infants = 10.0 to 14.0 g/dL Children = increase to adult		
H. Proper disposal and disinfection		
1. Disposed of all sharps in biohazard sharps containers.		
2. Disposed of all other regulated medical waste in biohazard bags.		
3. Disinfected test area and instruments according to OSHA guidelines.		
4. Sanitized hands after removing gloves.		
Totals Counts per Column		

Patient Name: _____

Patient Chart Entry: (Include when, what, why, any additional information, and the signature of the person charting.)

_____

_____

_____

Procedure 5.3: Hematocrit: General Procedure

Person evaluated _____   Date _____

Evaluated by _____

Outcome goal	Perform FDA-approved CLIA-waived hematocrit test following the most current OSHA safety guidelines and applying the correct quality control
Conditions	Supplies required: - Plastic capillary pipettes with anticoagulant - Sealant clay (e.g., Critoseal) or self-sealing capillary pipettes - Liquid controls: high and low - Gloves, gown, alcohol, gauze, and lancets - Hematocrit centrifuge with built-in reader or variable reader
Standards	Required time: 15 minutes Performance time: _____ Total possible points = _____ Points earned = _____
Evaluation Rubric Codes: **S** = Satisfactory, meets standard **U** = Unsatisfactory, fails to meet standard	
NOTE: Steps marked with an asterisk (*) are critical to achieve required competency.	

Preparation: Preanalytical Phase	Scores	
	S	**U**
A. Test information		
- Manufacturer: **Adams Readocrit (or other)**		
- Proper storage of pipettes and sealant (e.g., temperature, light): **room temperature**		
- Expiration date **(2 years or 30 days after opened)**		
- Package insert or test flow chart available: _____ yes ____ no		
B. Specimen information		
- Type of specimen: **capillary blood or venous blood in EDTA tube**		
- Specimen testing device: **two capillary tubes filled at least halfway**		
C. Personal protective equipment: **gloves, gown, face shield**		
D. Assembled all equipment, sanitized hands, and applied personal protective equipment		

Procedure: Analytical Phase	Scores	
	S	**U**
E. Performed/observed quality control		
1. Quantitative testing controls		
- **HemataCHEK reference control**		
- Control levels: high _____ low _____ normal _____		
F. Perform patient test		
1. Collected two heparin anticoagulated capillary tubes with blood from a finger or an EDTA tube of blood.		
- Held the capillary tube in a horizontal position or slightly tilted down to allow capillary action to pull the blood into the tube, as shown in Fig. A in the textbook.		
- Avoided allowing bubbles into specimen, and filled exactly to the line if using a built-in centrifuge scale or at least ½ full if using a variable reader.		

	Scores	
2. Sealed one end by pressing and turning in sealant [Fig. E] or tipped blood in the safety tube allowing the blood to make contact with thepresealed end of the tube [Fig. F] and then held the tube in a vertical position with the blood in contact with the sealant for 15 seconds.		
3. Placed the two tubes opposite each other with their clay ends toward the outside of the hematocrit centrifuge to create a balanced centrifuge (Fig. G).		
4. Locked the cover firmly against the capillary tubes to prevent breaking, and centrifuged for 5 minutes.		
5. Used the built-in scale (Fig. B) or the variable scales (Figures C and D) to adjust the total volume (starting where the clay meets the cells and where the plasma meets the air at the top); determined the percentage of the total volume.		
6. Depending on the hematocrit reader directions, located where the "RED CELL/PLASMA" interface could be seen, and determined the % of red cells in both specimens.		
7. Checked results of both capillary readings to see if they were within 2% of each other, and recorded the average of the two tubes.		
*Accurate Results _____ Instructor Confirmation _____		

Follow-up: Postanalytical Phase	Scores	
	S	U
*G. Proper documentation		
1. On control log _____ yes _____ no		
2. On patient log _____ yes _____ no		
3. Documented on patient chart (see below)		
4. Identified critical values and took appropriate steps to notify physician - Hematocrit expected values: Men = 42% to 52% Women = 36% to 48% Infants = 32% to 38% Children = increase to adult levels		
H. Proper disposal and disinfection		
1. Disposed of all sharps in biohazard sharps containers.		
2. Disposed of all other regulated medical waste in biohazard bags.		
3. Disinfected test area and instruments according to OSHA guidelines.		
4. Sanitized hands after removing gloves.		
Totals Counts per Column		

Patient Name: _____

Patient Chart Entry: (Include when, what, why, any additional information, and the signature of the person charting.)

_____

_____

_____

Procedure 5.4: Hematocrit: HemataSTAT Method

Person evaluated _____   Date _____

Evaluated by _____

Outcome goal	To perform FDA-approved CLIA-waived hematocrit test following the most current OSHA safety guidelines and applying the correct quality control
Conditions	Supplies required: - Plastic capillary pipettes with anticoagulant - Sealant clay (e.g., Critoseal) - Liquid controls: high and low - Gloves, gown, alcohol, gauze, and lancets
Standards	Required time: 15 minutes Performance time: _____ Total possible points = _____ Points earned = _____

Evaluation Rubric Codes:
S = Satisfactory, meets standard   **U** = Unsatisfactory, fails to meet standard

NOTE: Steps marked with an asterisk (*) are critical to achieve required competency.

Preparation: Preanalytical Phase	Scores	
	S	**U**
A. Test information		
- Kit or instrument method: **HemataSTAT II**		
- Manufacturer: **Separation Technology, Inc. (STI)**		
- Proper storage (e.g., temperature, light): **room temperature**		
- Expiration date **(2 years or 30 days after opened)**		
- Package insert or test flow chart available: _____ yes _____ no		
B. Specimen information		
- Type of specimen: **capillary blood or venous blood in EDTA tube**		
- Specimen testing device: **two capillary tubes filled at least halfway**		
C. Personal protective equipment: **gloves, gown, face shield**		
D. Assembled all equipment, sanitized hands, and applied personal protective equipment.		

Procedure: Analytical Phase	Scores	
	S	**U**
E. Performed/observed quality control		
1. Quantitative testing controls		
- **HemataCHEK reference control**		
- Control levels: high _____ low _____ normal _____		
F. Perform patient test		
1. Followed proper steps (from test flow chart).		
2. Collected whole blood into capillary tubes and sealed one end by pressing and turning in sealant and then tapped the sealed end.		
3. Inserted the sealed end of capillary tube into the HemataSTAT rotor tube holder.		
4. Closed centrifuge lid, locked latch, and pressed "RUN" to spin for 60 seconds.		

105

5. Waited for beeps, then unlocked latch and opened lid.		
6. Moved slider and sealed end of capillary tube to far left side of reader tray and rotated tube so entire "RED CELL/PLASMA" diagonal interface could be seen.		
7. Pressed "ENT" to read tube.		
8. Moved the slider black line to "SEALANT/RED CELL" interface and pressed "ENT."		
9. Moved the slider black line to "RED CELL/PLASMA" interface and pressed "ENT."		
10. Moved slider black line to "PLASMA/AIR" interface and pressed "ENT."		
11. Noted test result.		
12. Repeated steps 4 to 9 with second tube.		
- Result must be within 2% agreement of first reading.		
- Recorded the average of the two readings.		
*Accurate Results _____ **Instructor Confirmation** _____		

Follow-up: Postanalytical Phase	Scores	
	S	U
*G. Proper documentation		
1. On control log _____ yes _____ no		
2. On patient log _____ yes _____ no		
3. Documented on patient chart (see below)		

4. Identified critical values and took appropriate steps to notify physician.
  - Hematocrit expected values:
    Men = 42% to 52%
    Women = 36% to 48%
    Infants = 32% to 38%
    Children = increase to adult levels		

H. Proper disposal and disinfection		
1. Disposed of all sharps in biohazard sharps containers.		
2. Disposed of all other regulated medical waste in biohazard bags.		
3. Disinfected test area and instruments according to OSHA guidelines.		
4. Sanitized hands after removing gloves.		
Totals Counts per Column		

Patient Name: _____

Patient Chart Entry: (Include when, what, why, any additional information, and the signature of the person charting.)

_____

_____

_____

Procedure 5.5: ESR: SEDIPLAST System Procedure

Person evaluated _____   Date _____

Evaluated by _____

Outcome goal	To perform FDA-approved ESR waived test following the most current OSHA safety guidelines and applying the correct quality control
Conditions	Supplies needed: - Plastic Westergren pipette graduated from 0 to 200 mm - SEDIPLAST vials with citrate diluent - Westergren rack for holding the pipettes - Disposal transfer pipette - Timer - Gloves, gown, face shield
Standards	Required time: 70 minutes Performance time: _____ Total possible points = _____ Points earned = _____
Evaluation Rubric Codes: **S** = Satisfactory, meets standard **U** = Unsatisfactory, fails to meet standard	
NOTE: Steps marked with an asterisk (*) are critical to achieve required competency.	

Preparation: Preanalytical Phase	Scores	
	S	U
A. Test information		
- Kit or instrument method: **SEDIPLAST**		
- Manufacturer: **Polymedco, Inc.**		
- Proper storage (e.g., temperature, light): **room temperature**		
- Lot number on package: _____		
- Expiration date: _____		
- Package insert or test flow chart available: _____ yes_____ no		
B. Personal protective equipment: **gloves, gown, face shield**		
C. Proper specimen used for test		
- Type of specimen: **fresh EDTA whole blood that has been stored at room temperature for less than 2 hours or refrigerated blood up to 6 hours**		
- Specimen testing device: **SEDIPLAST vial and pipette**		
D. Assembled all equipment, sanitized hands, and applied personal protective equipment.		

Procedure: Analytical Phase	Scores	
	S	U
E. Performed/observed quality control methods: not applicable.		
F. Performed patient test		
1. Removed stopper on vial and filled the vial with blood to indicated mark with a disposable transfer pipette (0.8 mL of blood needed).		
2. Replaced vial stopper and inverted vial several times to mix.		
3. Placed vial in SEDIPLAST rack on a level surface free of vibrations and jarring.		

Chapter **5 Hematology**

	Scores	

4. Pressed the disposable SEDIPLAST pipette gently through the stopper with a twisting motion and continued to press until the pipette rested on the bottom of the vial (the pipette auto-zeros the blood, and any excess flows into the closed reservoir compartment at the top of the pipette).

5. Set the timer for 1 hour, and let specimen stand undisturbed.

6. After 1 hour, read the numeric results of the ESR (used the scale at the top of the pipette to measure the distance from the top of the plasma to the top of the red blood cells).

*Accurate Results _____ **Instructor Confirmation** _____

Follow-up: Postanalytical Phase	Scores	
	S	U
*G. Proper documentation		
1. On patient log _____ yes _____ no		
2. Documented on patient chart (see below).		

3. Identified critical values, and took appropriate steps to notify physician.
     - ESR expected values:
      Men $<$ 50 years old = 0 to 15 mm/hr
      Men $>$ 50 years old = 0 to 20 mm/hr
      Women $<$ 50 years old = 0 to 20 mm/hr
      Women $>$ 50 years old = 0 to 30 mm/hr		

H. Proper disposal and disinfection		
1. Disposed of all sharps in biohazard sharps containers.		
2. Disposed of all other regulated medical waste in biohazard bags.		
3. Disinfected test area and instruments according to OSHA guidelines.		
4. Sanitized hands after removing gloves.		
Totals Counts per Column		

Patient Name: _____

Patient Chart Entry: (Include when, what, why, any additional information, and the signature of the person charting.)

_____

_____

_____

Procedure 5.6: ESR: Streck 30-minute Procedure

Person evaluated _____   Date _____

Evaluated by _____

Outcome goal	To perform FDA-approved CLIA-waived ESR test following the most current OSHA safety guidelines and applying the correct quality control
Conditions	Supplies needed: - Black Streck citrate tubes and venipuncture supplies - Streck rack - Timer - Personal protective equipment
Standards	Required time: 40 minutes Performance time: _____ Total possible points = _____ Points earned = _____

Evaluation Rubric Codes:
S = Satisfactory, meets standard   **U** = Unsatisfactory, fails to meet standard

NOTE: Steps marked with an asterisk (*) are critical to achieve required competency.

Preparation: Preanalytical Phase	Scores	
	S	**U**
A. Test information		
- Kit or instrument method: **Streck ESR**		
- Manufacturer: STRECK		
- Proper storage (e.g., temperature, light): **room temperature**		
- Lot number on package: _____		
- Expiration date: _____		
- Package insert or test flow chart available: _____ yes_____ no		
B. Personal protective equipment: **gloves, gown, face shield**		
C. Proper specimen used for test		
■ Collect the blood in a black topped Streck citrate tube making sure to push and hold the tube stopper firmly against the holder.		
■ Position the tube at an angle that allows the blood stream to hit the wall before mixing with the citrate solution to minimize the formation of blood foam.		
■ The blood will stop flowing near the indicated line on the bottom of the Streck tube's label.		
■ Immediately remove the tube and tilt 8 to 10 times.		
■ (Note: If using a butterfly needle, a waste tube will be needed to clear the air from the tubing.) Blood from an EDTA tube may also be used. It will need to be transferred into the black tube. In both cases, the blood must be mixed immediately after drawing.		

Procedure: Analytical Phase	Scores	
	S	U
D. Allow the liquid controls and the labeled blood specimen to come to room temperature while mixing thoroughly on a rotating blood mixer for 15 minutes.		
E. Performed patient test		
■ Place the ESR vacuum tube in any free position in the ESR-10 Manual Rack with the stopper in the upright position.		
■ Each tube position is marked with a red circle numbered 1 through 10.		
■ Align the tube so that the bottom of the liquid's curved meniscus is in line with the zero position on the measuring scale.		
■ Note: Do not adjust the position of the tube by pulling on the stopper. Allow the tube to settle in an undisturbed, vertical position for 30 minutes.		
■ After 30 minutes, record the numerical value at the top of the column of sedimented erythrocytes. Report the result as mm/hr, modified Westergren method.		
*Accurate Results _____ Instructor Confirmation _____		

Follow-up: Postanalytical Phase	Scores	
	S	U
*F. Proper documentation		
1. On patient log _____ yes _____ no		
2. Documented on patient chart (see below).		
3. Identified critical values, and took appropriate steps to notify physician. - ESR expected values: Men < 50 years old = 0 to 15 mm/hr Men > 50 years old = 0 to 20 mm/hr Women < 50 years old = 0 to 20 mm/hr Women > 50 years old = 0 to 30 mm/hr		
G. Proper disposal and disinfection		
1. Disposed of all sharps in biohazard sharps containers.		
2. Disposed of all other regulated medical waste in biohazard bags.		
3. Disinfected test area and instruments according to OSHA guidelines.		
4. Sanitized hands after removing gloves.		
Totals Counts per Column		

Patient Name: _____

Patient Chart Entry: (Include when, what, why, any additional information, and the signature of the person charting.)

_____

_____

_____

Procedure 5.7: Prothrombin Time/INR CoaguChek Method

CAAHEP COMPETENCIES: I.P11, II.P3

ABHES COMPETENCIES: 9.i, 9.m, 10.a, 10.b

Person evaluated _____   Date _____

Evaluated by _____

Outcome goal	To perform an FDA-approved CLIA-waived coagulation test to determine prothrombin time/INR following the most current OSHA safety guidelines and applying correct quality control
Conditions	Supplies needed: - Gloves, fluid-impermeable lab coat - Alcohol, gauze, and bandage for capillary puncture site care - CoaguChek lancet - CoaguChek test strip container and its code chip - CoaguChek XS PT test monitor - Package insert or flow chart with directions - Biohazard sharps container
Standards	Required time: 10 minutes Performance time: _____ Total possible points = _____ Points earned = _____
Evaluation Rubric Codes: **S** = Satisfactory, meets standard **U** = Unsatisfactory, fails to meet standard	
NOTE: Steps marked with an asterisk (*) are critical to achieve required competency.	

Preparation: Preanalytical Phase	Scores	
	S	U
A. Test information		
- Kit or instrument method: **CoaguChek**		
- Manufacturer: **ROCHE**		
- Proper storage (e.g., temperature, light): **foil-pouched test strips are refrigerated and must come to room temperature before opening**		
- Expiration date: _____		
- Lot number on strip: _____		
- Package insert or test flow chart available: _____ yes _____ no		
B. Personal protective equipment: **gloves, gown, face shield**		
C. Proper specimen used for test		
- Type of specimen: **finger stick blood from a finger that has been warmed and gently massaged**		
D. Assembled all equipment, (Fig. A), sanitized hands, and applied personal protective equipment.		

Procedure: Analytical Phase	Scores	
	S	U
E. Performed/observed quality control		
- Quantitative testing controls		
- Calibration check: If you are using test strips from a new, unopened container, you must change the test strip code chip. The three-number code on the test strip container must match the three-number code on the code strip. To install the code chip, follow the instructions in the Code Chip section of the *User Manual*.		
- Control levels: **level I control, and level II control**		
F. Performed patient test		
1. Place the meter on a flat surface so that it will not vibrate or move during testing.		
2. Identify the patient using two identifiers (such as having them spell their last name and state their birth date, and/or show a picture identification), then explain the procedure to the patient.."	*	
3. Examine the fingers and choose the site to be used to obtain the blood sample.		
4. Prepare the site for a good drop of blood by doing the following prior to lancing the finger:		
- Warm the hand by placing it under the arm, using a hand warmer, and/or washing the hand in warm water.		
- Have the patient hold his or her arm down to the side so that the hand is below the waist.		
- Massage the palm of the hand toward base of the finger and toward the tip until the fingertip has increased color.		
- NOTE: If needed, immediately after lancing, gently squeeze the finger from its base to encourage blood flow.		
5. When you are ready to test, remove one test strip from the container and **immediately close the container. Make sure it seals tightly. Do not open the container or touch the test strips with wet hands or wet gloves.**		
6. Insert test strip as far as you can into the meter. This powers the meter ON.		
7. Press "Patient Test" on the meter display. The meter warms the test strip. Then the meter begins a countdown. You have 180 seconds to apply a blood sample to the test strip.		
8. Disinfect the finger with alcohol and wipe dry. Perform the finger stick.		
9. Hold the incised finger very close to the target (clear area of the test strip) and apply one drop of blood to the top or side of the target area (Fig. B) and wait until you hear the beep. **You must apply a hanging drop of blood to the test strip within 15 seconds of lancing the finger. Do not add more blood. Do not touch or remove the test strip while the test is in progress.** The flashing blood drop symbol changes to an hourglass symbol when the meter detects a sufficient sample.	*	
10. The result appears in approximately 1 minute. (Fig. C) The results may be displayed in three ways: the International Normalized Ratio (INR), a prothrombin time (PT) in seconds, or as %Quick (a unit used mainly in Europe).		
11. Read and recorded the INR and PT from the digital screen.	*	
*Accurate Results INR _____ PT _____ Instructor Confirmation _____		

Follow-up: Postanalytical Phase	Scores	
	S	U
*G. Proper documentation		
1. On patient log _____ yes _____ no		
2. Documented on patient chart (see below).		
3. Identified critical values and took appropriate steps to notify physician.		
ProTime expected values for normal and therapeutic whole blood: <table><tr><td></td><td>INR</td><td>PT (in seconds)</td></tr><tr><td>**Normal**</td><td>0.8–1.2</td><td>*6.5 to 11.9 seconds for INR method</td></tr><tr><td>**Low Anticoagulation Therapy**</td><td>1.5–2.0</td><td>Varies with method used</td></tr><tr><td>**Moderate Anticoagulation Therapy**</td><td>2.0–3.0</td><td>Varies with method used</td></tr><tr><td>**High Anticoagulation Therapy**</td><td>3.0–4.0</td><td>Varies with method used</td></tr></table> *Laboratory reports and manufacturers must supply their own reference ranges along with each patient's results. This is because different methodologies may create different reference ranges as well as different units of measurement.		
*H. Proper disposal and disinfection		
1. Disposed of all sharps in biohazard sharps containers.		
2. Disposed of all other regulated medical waste in biohazard bags.		
3. Disinfected test area and instruments according to OSHA guidelines.		
4. Sanitized hands after removing gloves.		
Totals Counts per Column		

Patient Name: _____

Patient Chart Entry: (Include when, what, why, any additional information, and the signature of the person charting.)

_____

_____

_____

6 | Chemistry

VOCABULARY REVIEW

Match each definition with the correct term.

_____ 1. Chemicals that produce specific changes in other substances without being changed themselves

_____ 2. Groups of tests providing information on particular organs or body metabolism

_____ 3. Glucose permanently changed the hemoglobin molecule within red blood cells

_____ 4. Abnormal fat levels in the blood

_____ 5. Formation of plaque along the inside walls of blood vessels

_____ 6. Sugars and starches

_____ 7. Sugar in the urine

_____ 8. Cholesterol derived from the diet

_____ 9. Man-made hydrogenated fats

_____ 10. Elevated blood sugar

_____ 11. Fats and proteins that are able to convert to glucose if necessary

_____ 12. Electrolytes consisting of positively or negatively charged particles

_____ 13. Excessively high blood insulin levels

_____ 14. Hormone produced by the pancreas to lower blood glucose

_____ 15. Diagnosis based on the patient's initial signs and symptoms

_____ 16. Excessive fat in blood, giving a milky appearance in the plasma

_____ 17. Condition of excessive ketones in the blood causing an acid condition

_____ 18. Hormone produced by the pancreas to raise blood glucose

_____ 19. Stored form of glucose especially found in muscles and the liver

_____ 20. Cholesterol manufactured in the liver

_____ 21. Final, confirmed diagnosis based on clinical signs and symptoms and the results of diagnostic tests

A. endogenous cholesterol
B. glycogen
C. exogenous cholesterol
D. catalysts
E. hyperinsulinemia
F. glycosylated HgbA1c
G. hyperlipidemia
H. insulin
I. glucagon
J. *trans* fats
K. ions
L. glycosuria
M. atherosclerosis
N. panels
O. dyslipidemia
P. carbohydrates
Q. definitive diagnosis
R. hyperglycemia
S. clinical diagnosis
T. ketoacidosis
U. noncarbohydrate energy sources

114

Chapter **6 Chemistry**

FUNDAMENTAL CONCEPTS

22. Provide the missing information in the plasma flow chart (see Fig. 6.1 in the textbook).

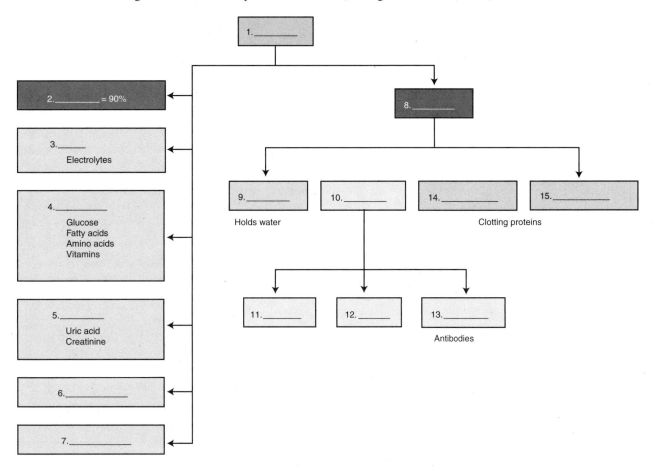

23. Match the categories of chemicals found in plasma with their associated substances (see Fig. 6.1 in the textbook).

_____ clotting proteins

_____ nutrients

_____ hormones

_____ proteins

_____ wastes

_____ salts

_____ gamma globulins

_____ enzymes

_____ the three globulins

A. albumins and globulins

B. electrolytes

C. alpha, beta, and gamma

D. catalysts

E. glucose, amino acids, and fatty acids

F. antibodies

G. thyroid and pituitary glands

H. prothrombin and fibrinogen

I. urea, uric acid, creatinine

Chapter **6 Chemistry**

24. Describe the three layers that are formed when the gold "SST" tube has been centrifuged. Which layer is used for chemistry testing? (HINT: See Fig. 6.2)

_____

_____

_____

25. Refer to the sample requisition in the textbook (see Fig. 6.3), and identify what color tube top to use for each of the following tests:

prothrombin time _____ BUN _____

lipid panel _____ CBC w/Diff _____

renal function panel _____ mono test _____

26. When prothrombin and fibrinogen are removed from plasma, the remaining liquid is referred to as _____

_____.

27. Define the following glucose-related abbreviations.

A1c _____ IGT _____

FBG _____ NIDDM _____

FPG _____ OGTT _____

GTT _____ 2-hr PP _____

IDDM _____

28. How is glucose metabolized in the following locations?

Body cells _____

Liver _____

Muscles _____

Adipose tissue _____

29. List the two ways insulin lowers the level of blood glucose.

_____

_____

30. List the two ways glucagon raises the level of blood glucose.

_____

_____

31. What two lifestyle changes can a prediabetic patient make to prevent or delay the development of type 2 diabetes?

_____

_____

32. List three beneficial functions of cholesterol.

_____

_____

_____

33. List the two dietary fats that elevate the bad type of cholesterol (LDL).

_____

_____

34. Define the following lipid-related abbreviations.

HDL _____

LDL _____

TC/HDL ratio _____

VLDL _____

35. List two dietary fats that elevate the good type of cholesterol (HDL).

_____

_____

36. Why is LDL cholesterol referred to as "lousy" cholesterol and HDL referred to as "healthy" cholesterol?

_____

_____

37. Physicians are likely to be more interested in which of the following as a predictive indicator of future myocardial infarction?

    a. Cholesterol value

    b. LDL value

    c. Cholesterol/HDL ratio

    d. HDL value

38. People who exercise regularly, maintain normal weight, and eat mostly unsaturated fats will probably increase their level of

    a. HDL

    b. LDL

    c. Albumin

    d. Glucose

39. When testing for triglycerides, the patient should refrain from alcohol for _____ days before testing and fast for _____ hours before the test.

PROCEDURES: CLIA-WAIVED CHEMISTRY TESTS

40. What is the purpose of *calibrating* a blood chemistry analyzer? (Hint: Think of the calibrator checks when running the Cholestech.)

_____

_____

41. Complete the following tasks.

   A. List three reasons or causes why a liquid control would fall outside its designated range.

   _____

   _____

   _____

   B. Using the monthly Levy-Jennings chart at the end of this chapter, record the following control settings and daily results for the normal liquid glucose control (NOTE: On days 13 and 17 the controls were repeated because the first result was out of control):

   Reference range for control = 96-136 mg/dL
       +2 standard deviations = 136
       +1 standard deviation = 126
   Mean = 116
       −1 standard deviation = 106
       −2 standard deviations = 96

Daily Results

1. 118	7. 108	13. 137	17. repeat 110	23. 120	29. 114
2. 114	8. 114	13. repeat 125	18. 99	24. 114	30. 115
3. 113	9. 120	14. 117	19. 105	25. 133	31. 116
4. 104	10. 118	15. 106	20. 105	26. 123	
5. 101	11. 120	16. 114	21. 110	27. 130	
6. 100	12. 130	17. 94	22. 118	28. 116	

   C. When looking at the chart, were any of the Westgard Rules below broken? (Circle the numbers that apply.)

   Should you continue using the monitor and/or strips? _____
   1. Both levels of control results were outside the manufacturer's reference range (if running a normal and high control). *Note:* This rule does not apply because we are monitoring only one control.
   2. The same control level fell outside of the reference range in two successive runs.
   3. One of the controls fell outside of the plus or minus 1 standard deviation in four successive runs.
   4. One of the controls consistently fell above the mean value or consistently fell below the mean value for 10 consecutive runs.

   D. (OPTIONAL) If available, chart the class results for the liquid glucose control on the second Levy-Jennings chart found at the end of this chapter, and analyze the results based on the Westgard Rules.

42. List three foods that the patient should avoid 2 days before collecting a fecal specimen used for the occult blood test. What is the name of the fecal occult test that does not require eliminating these foods?

   _____

   _____

   _____

43. What is the name of the home fecal occult blood test for which the patient places the test paper directly into the toilet? _____ If the test area of the paper turns green or blue, is the result positive or negative?

   _____

44. Label the supplies and equipment for the test kit method for A_{1c} (see Procedure 6.2 in the textbook). What is the supply item that must be used for all 20 tests in the kit? _____ May that item be used with cartridges from another kit? _____

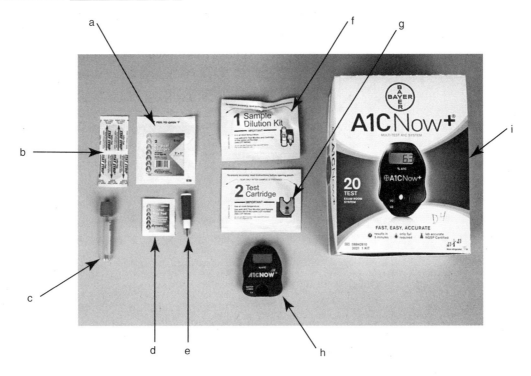

45. Label the Cholestech LDX equipment and supplies (see Procedure 6.3 in the textbook).

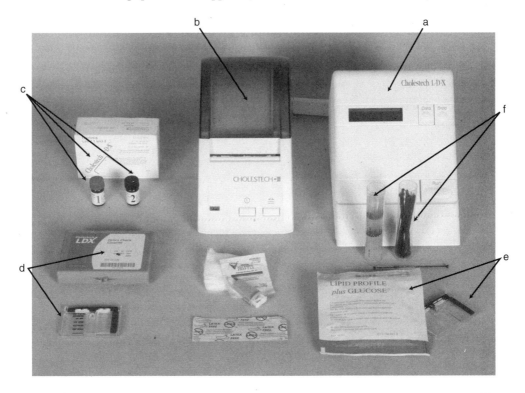

46. Label the ColoScreen III equipment and supplies (see Procedure 6.5 in the textbook).

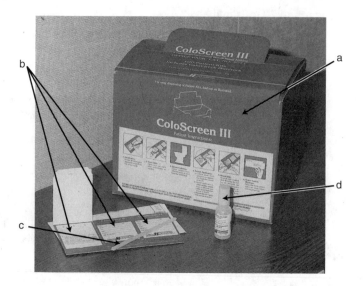

ADVANCED CONCEPTS

Match each procedural step and advanced concept term with the correct definition.

_____ 47. cation

_____ 48. galvanometer

_____ 49. reflectance photometry

_____ 50. troponins I and T

_____ 51. bilirubin

_____ 52. absorbance photometry

_____ 53. anion

_____ 54. i-STAT and Piccolo

_____ 55. transmittance photometry

_____ 56. calibration

_____ 57. occult

_____ 58. gout

_____ 59. myoglobin

A. Form of arthritis caused by accumulation of uric acid crystals in the synovial fluid
B. Hidden or not visible to the naked eye
C. Heme-containing, oxygen-binding protein found in muscles
D. Positively charged ion
E. "Optics check" or setting to ensure the analyzer's optics are working correctly with the testing devices
F. Measurement of the amount of light passing through the solution
G. CLIA-waived chemistry analyzers
H. Heart-specific indicators of a recent myocardial infarction
I. Measurement of the light that reflects off of the specimen
J. Measurement of the amount of light the solution absorbs
K. Waste product from the breakdown of hemoglobin
L. Negatively charged ion
M. Instrument capable of measuring the intensity of light

60. List eight critical chemistry tests that are typically monitored during a medical emergency. (Hint: See i-STAT test.)

_____   _____

_____   _____

_____   _____

_____   _____

61. Match each chemistry panel with its representative group of tests.

_____ cardiac panel   A. Twelve or more tests

_____ liver, hepatic panel   B. BUN, creatinine, uric acid

_____ kidney, renal panel   C. Sodium, potassium, chloride

_____ lipid panel   D. Bilirubin, AST, ALT, ALP, LD, GGT

_____ thyroid panel   E. Troponins I and T, CK, LD, ALT, myoglobin

_____ metabolic panel   F. TSH, T_4, T_3 uptake

_____ electrolyte panel   G. TC, HDL, LDL, triglycerides

62. Match the analytes with the medical condition or organ that is being monitored.

_____ uric acid   A. Diabetes

_____ cholesterol   B. Hepatitis or liver function

_____ BUN   C. Gout

_____ glucose   D. Coronary artery disease and atherosclerosis

_____ bilirubin   E. Nephritis or kidney function

Chemistry Abbreviations

63. Using the alphabetical list of abbreviations at the beginning of Chapter 6 in the textbook, identify the six enzyme abbreviations routinely tested for tissue or organ damage. (Hint: Remember enzymes have the suffix -*ase*.) Then identify two organs or the diseases that are associated with each enzyme. Use the categorical chart of blood chemistry analytes (see Table 6-3 in the textbook) at the end of the chapter to locate the diseases.

Enzyme Abbreviation	Enzyme	Affected Organs and Associated Diseases
1.		
2.		
3.		
4.		
5.		
6.		

64. List the four electrolyte abbreviations found at the beginning of the chapter and state whether they are cations or anions. (Hint: They have positive or negative charges after their abbreviations.)

Electrolyte Abbreviation	Electrolyte	Cation/Anion (+/−)
1.		
2.		
3.		
4.		

121

Procedure 6.1: Glucometer Procedure

Person evaluated _____   Date _____

Evaluated by _____   Score _____

Outcome goal	To perform FDA-approved CLIA-waived glucose test following the most current OSHA safety guidelines and applying correct quality control
Conditions	Supplies needed: - CONTOUR monitor - Coded test strip and liquid control - Lancet, alcohol, gauze, bandage - Personal protective equipment
Standards	Required time: 5 minutes Performance time: _____ Total possible points = _____ Points earned = _____
Evaluation Rubric Codes: **S** = Satisfactory, meets standard **U** = Unsatisfactory, fails to meet standard	
NOTE: Steps marked with an asterisk (*) are critical to achieve required competency.	

Preparation	Scores	
	S	U
A. Test information		
- Kit or instrument method: **Contour**		
- Manufacturer: **Bayer**		
- Proper storage (e.g., temperature, light): **test strips and controls are stored at room temperature**		
- Expiration date _____		
- Lot #: _____ Calibration #: _____		
- Package insert or test flow chart available: yes _____ no _____		
B. Personal protective equipment: **gloves, gown, biohazard container**		
C. Specimen information		
- Type of specimen: **fasting, 2-hour postprandial, or random specimen**		
- Specimen source: **capillary blood or lavender-topped vacuum tube** (Note: gray-topped tubes are not used for this method.)		
- Specimen testing device: **coded test strips**		
D. Assembled all the above, sanitized hands, and applied personal protective equipment.		

Procedure: Analytical Phase	Scores	
	S	U
E. Performed/observed quantitative quality control		
- Calibration check is done automatically when each strip is inserted.		
- (*Note:* Older versions need to set the code number on the meter based on the test strip number.)		
- Control levels: Normal _____ High _____		
- (Manufacturer recommendation: Run normal control with each new batch of strips, with each new operator, and then weekly.)		

	S	U
F. Performed patient test		
1. Turned on meter by inserting test strip's end with the contact bars.		
2. Stuck finger and *touched the end of the strip into the drop* of blood, allowing the blood to flow ("sip") into the strip without interruption.		
- Did **not** smear or place blood on top or bottom of strip.		
3. When beep was heard, removed the glucometer and strip away from drop of blood.		
4. Result displayed on the screen.		
*Accurate Results _____ **Instructor Confirmation** _____		

Follow-up: Postanalytical Phase	Scores	
	S	U
*G. Proper documentation		
1. On control log: _____ yes _____ no		
2. On patient log: _____ yes _____ no		
3. Documentation on patient chart (see following page)		
H. Identified "critical values" and took appropriate steps to notify physician		

    - Expected ranges for glucose based on ADA recommendations

Fasting	2-Hour	Postprandial (After Drinking a Glucose-Rich Beverage)
Normal	< 100 mg/dL	140 mg/dL
Prediabetes	T body: 100-125 mg/dL	140-199 mg/dL
Diabetes	≥ 126 mg/dL	≥ 200 mg/dL

	S	U
I. Proper disposal and disinfection		
1. Disposed of all sharps in biohazard sharps containers.		
2. Disposed of all other regulated medical waste in biohazard bags.		
3. Disinfected test area and instruments according to OSHA guidelines.		
4. Sanitized hands after removing gloves.		
Total Points per Column		

Patient Name: _____

Patient Chart Entry: (Include when, what, how, why, any additional information, and the signature of the person charting.)

_____

_____

_____

Procedure 6.2: A₁c NOW+ Glycosylated Hemoglobin Procedure

Person evaluated _____ Date _____

Evaluated by _____ Score _____

Outcome goal	To perform FDA-approved glycosylated hemoglobin A_{1c} waived test following the most current OSHA safety guidelines and applying the correct quality control
Conditions	Supplies needed: - Gauze, bandage, alcohol swab - Lancet for capillary blood sample or heparin tube with venous blood sample - Sample dilution kit containing capillary tube collector and sampler body - Test cartridge - A1c monitor programmed to work only with the 20 cartridges in the kit - Personal protective equipment
Standards	Required time: 5 minutes Performance time: _____ Total possible points = _____ Points earned = _____
Evaluation Rubric Codes: **S** = Satisfactory, meets standard **U** = Unsatisfactory, fails to meet standard	
NOTE: Steps marked with an asterisk (*) are critical to achieve required competency.	

Preparation: Preanalytical Phase	Scores S	Scores U
A. Test information		
- Kit or instrument method: **A1cNOW1 test kit method**		
- Manufacturer: **Bayer**		
- Proper storage (e.g., temperature, light): **Foil-wrapped cartridges and kits are refrigerated. Allow 1 hour to warm to room temperature.**		
- Expiration date: _____		
- Lot # of cartridges: _____		
- Package insert or test flow chart available: _____ yes _____ no		
B. Personal protective equipment: **gloves, gown, face shield**		
C. Proper specimen used for test		
- Use only **fresh capillary blood** or venous whole blood collected in a **heparin (green top) tube**. Venous blood can be used only if the tube is less than 1 week old and has been refrigerated during that time. Ensure blood in heparin tube is well mixed and at room temperature.		
- Specimen testing device: microcapillary tube provided in kit. After the glass capillary tube has been filled with the specimen, the analysis must begin within 5 minutes.		
D. Assembled all the above and ensured they were at the same temperature (within 18°C to 28°C), sanitized hands, and applied personal protective equipment		

Procedure: Analytical Phase	Scores	
	S	U
E. Performed/observed quantitative quality control		
- Optics check: Each box of test kits has already set its optics (make sure code on cartridge matches the code on monitor, but do not open until just before inserting into monitor).		
- Control levels: _____normal abnormal _____		
F. Performed patient test		
1. Removed the blood collector from the foil #1 sampler dilution kit and gently touched the tip of the capillary tube that was attached to the holder into the small drop of blood from the finger stick or the venous blood drop on the slide.		
- The blood should fill the small glass capillary tube without touching the plastic holder.		
2. Wiped the sides of the capillary tube with tissue.		
3. Fully inserted the capillary holder into the sampler body that also came from the #1 sampler dilution kit (pushed together and twisted until the holder and sampler body snapped into place).		
4. Mixed sample with the dilution by tilting 6 to 8 times; stood the sampler on the table.		
5. Opened the #2 test cartridge foil package and performed the following within 2 minutes:		
- Clicked the cartridge into the monitor that came in the same kit box; checked code numbers, which must match.		
- While the monitor indicated "WAIT," prepared the sample by removing the base.		
- Did not add the sample until the monitor indicated "SMPL."		
- Pushed sampler down onto the white well of the cartridge.		
- The monitor was on a level surface and was not moved until the test was complete.		
6. After several minutes, the monitor indicated "QCOK," followed by the test result and by the number of tests left in the kit.		
7. Recorded the results from the display and reported to the physician.		
*Accurate Results _____ Instructor Confirmation _____		

Follow-up: Postanalytical Phase	Scores	
	S	U
*G. Proper documentation		
1. Control logs: _____ yes _____ no		
2. Patient log: _____ yes _____ no		
3. Documentation on patient chart (see following page).		
4. Identified critical values and took appropriate steps to notify physician.		
- Expected values:		

Nondiabetics	3%-6%
Controlled diabetics	6%-8%
Poorly controlled diabetics	20% or higher

Note: Because A_{1c} is also affected by the hemoglobin concentration, normal ranges should be determined by each laboratory to conform to the population being tested.

H. Proper disposal and disinfection		
1. Disposed of the cartridge in biohazard sharps containers, and returned monitor to the box for subsequent testing.		
2. Disposed of all other regulated medical waste in biohazard bags.		
3. Disinfected test area and instruments according to OSHA guidelines.		
4. Sanitized hands after removing gloves.		
Total Points per Column		

Patient Name: _____

Patient Chart Entry: (Include when, what, how, why, any additional information, and the signature of the person charting.)

_____

_____

_____

Procedure 6.3: Cholestech Method of Measuring Lipids and Glucose

Person evaluated _____   Date _____

Evaluated by _____   Score _____

Outcome goal	To perform FDA-approved lipid profile waived test following the most current OSHA safety guidelines and applying the correct quality control.
Conditions	Supplies needed: - Optics check cassette - Level 1 and 2 liquid controls - Alcohol, gauze, and lancets or vacuum lithium heparin tubes - Capillary tubes and plungers for finger stick sample - Mini-Pet pipette and pipette tips for venipuncture sample - Personal protective equipment
Standards	Required time: 10 minutes Performance time: _____ Total possible points = _____ Points earned = _____

Evaluation Rubric Codes:
S = Satisfactory, meets standard   **U** = Unsatisfactory, fails to meet standard

NOTE: Steps marked with an asterisk (*) are critical to achieve required competency.

Preparation: Preanalytical Phase	Scores	
	S	U
A. Test information		
- Kit or instrument method: **Cholestech LDX Analyzer**		
- Manufacturer: **Cholestech Corporation**		
- Proper storage (e.g., temperature, light): **Foil-wrapped cassettes are refrigerated. They must return to room temperature before testing.**		
- Expiration date: _____		
- Cassette lot #: _____		
- Package insert or test flow chart available: _____ yes _____ no		
B. Personal protective equipment: **gloves, gown, biohazard containers**		
C. Specimen information		
- Patient preparation: **Fasting recommended for cholesterol. Triglyceride requires fasting and no alcohol consumption in previous 48 hours.**		
- Type of specimen: **capillary blood or lithium heparin (green top) tube only for venous blood**		
- Specimen testing device: **Cholestech capillary tube (once in tube, must be tested within 5 minutes)**		
D. Assembled all the above, sanitized hands, and applied personal protective equipment		

Procedure: Analytical Phase	Scores	
	S	U
E. Performed/observed quantitative quality control		
- Calibration check: **Run calibration cassette daily.**		
- Control levels: **Level 1, Level 2** (Use the mini-Pet pipettes provided by Cholestech)		

	S	
F. Performed patient test		
1. Allowed cassette to come to room temperature (at least 10 minutes before opening).		
2. Made sure analyzer was plugged in and warmed up.		
3. Removed cassette from its pouch and placed it on flat surface.		
- Held cassette by the short sides only.		
- Did not touch the black bar or the brown magnetic strip.		
4. Pressed RUN; the analyzer did a self-test, and the screen displayed "selftest running" and then "selftest OK."		
5. The cassette drawer opened, and the screen displayed "load cassette and press RUN."		
- Drawer remains open for 4 minutes, after which it closes with the message "System time-out: RUN to continue." If the RUN button is not pushed within 15 seconds, the drawer closes, and the screen goes blank. Press RUN again, allow to go through the self-test again, and proceed.		
6. Collected fresh capillary blood to the black line of the capillary tube with plunger inserted into the red end of the tube.		
- Or collected fresh venous whole blood with the Cholestech mini-Pet pipette.		
7. Placed whole blood sample into the test cassette sample well.		
- The finger stick sample must be put into the cassette within 5 minutes of collection or the blood will clot.		
8. *Immediately* placed cassette into the drawer of the analyzer.		
- Kept cassette level after the sample was applied.		
- The black reaction bar faced toward the analyzer.		
- The brown magnetic strip was on the right.		
9. Pressed RUN. The drawer closed, and the screen displayed "[test names]—running."		
10. When the test was completed, the analyzer beeped, and the screen displayed results at the same time the printer printed results. (Press DATA to display the calculated results of all tests on the screen if running a panel of tests.)		
*Accurate Results _____ **Instructor Confirmation** _____		

Follow-up: Postanalytical Phase	Scores	
	S	**U**
G. Proper documentation		
1. On control log: _____ yes _____ no		
2. On patient log: _____ yes _____ no		
3. Documented on patient chart (see below).		
4. Identified "critical values" and took appropriate steps to notify physician.		

Test	Desirable		
NCEP ATP III guidelines for lipid panels:			
Test	**Desirable**		
Total cholesterol (TC)	<200 mg/dL		
HDL cholesterol	>40 mg/dL		
LDL cholesterol	<130 mg/dL		
Triglycerides	**<150 mg/dL**		
TC/HDL ratio	**≤ 4.5**		
Glucose	**Fasting: 60-110 mg/dL**		
	Nonfasting: <160 mg/dL		
Alanine aminotransferase	**10-40 U/L**		
H. Proper disposal and disinfection			
1. Disposed of all sharps into biohazard sharps containers.			
2. Disposed of all other regulated medical waste into biohazard bags.			
3. Disinfected test area and instruments according to OSHA guidelines.			
4. Sanitized hands after removing gloves.			
Total Points per Column			

Patient Name: _____

Attach printed readout, or record results on the chart provided:

Test	Results	Desirable
Total cholesterol (TC)		<200 mg/dL
HDL cholesterol		>40 mg/dL
LDL cholesterol		<130 mg/dL
Triglycerides		<150 mg/dL
TC/HDL ratio		≤ 4.5
Other		
Glucose		Fasting: 60-110 mg/dL
		Nonfasting: <160 mg/dL

Procedure 6.4: i-STAT Chemistry Analyzer Procedure

Person evaluated _____   Date _____

Evaluated by _____   Score _____

Outcome goal	To perform FDA-approved i-STAT chemistry waived test following the most current OSHA safety guidelines and applying the correct quality control
Conditions	Supplies needed: - i-STAT 1 handheld, recharging dock, and printer - Ampule of Level 1 liquid control for i-STAT CHEM 8+ - i-STAT CHEM 8+ cartridges - Fresh blood collected in lithium heparin tubes (green top) - 1-mL plain syringe - Safety transfer device or safety tip - Personal protective equipment and biohazard container
Standards	Required time: 15 minutes Performance time: _____ Total possible points = _____ Points earned = _____

Evaluation Rubric Codes:
S = Satisfactory, meets standard   **U** = Unsatisfactory, fails to meet standard

NOTE: Steps marked with an asterisk (*) are critical to achieve required competency.

Preparation: Preanalytical Phase	Scores	
	S	**U**
A. Test information		
- Kit or instrument method: **i-STAT Chemistry Analyzer**		
- Manufacturer: **Abbott**		
- Proper storage (e.g., temperature, light): **Foil-wrapped cartridges and controls are refrigerated. They must return to room temperature before testing.**		
- Expiration date: _____		
- Scan cartridge lot #: _____		
- Package insert or test flow chart available: _____ yes _____no		
B. Personal protective equipment: **gloves, gown, biohazard containers**		
C. Specimen information		
- Patient preparation: **Collect blood, ensuring the 4-mL heparin tube fills completely and is mixed by tilting 10 times. Specimen should be tested within 10 minutes.**		
- Type of specimen: **Lithium heparin (green top) tube only for venous blood**		
- Specimen testing device: **A 1-mL syringe is used to remove the specimen from the green-topped vacuum tube and transfer the blood to the cartridge.**		
D. Assembled all the above, sanitized hands, and applied personal protective equipment.		

Procedure: Analytical Phase	Scores	
	S	U
E. Performed/observed quantitative quality control		
- Calibration check: **Use the simulator provided by i-STAT.**		
- Control level: **Level 1 ampule is provided by i-STAT.**		
F. Performed patient test		
1. Allowed cassette to come to room temperature (at least 10 minutes before opening).		
2. Keyed in operator and patient information into the handheld analyzer, followed by scanning the cartridge bar code until a beep was heard.		
3. *Within 10 minutes* of drawing a 4-mL specimen of blood into a vacuum tube, performed the following:		
- Mixed the specimen by tilting 10 times.		
- Connected a safety tip or safety transfer device to a 1-mL syringe.		
- Inverted the green-top tube with the specimen and pierced the green stopper with the syringe safety tip or the transfer device.		
- *Slowly* pulled back on the syringe plunger until it was about one half full; noted any air bubbles that entered syringe while transferring and did not push them back into specimen.		
- Disconnected syringe from vacuum tube and continued to hold it with tip pointed upward; held a gauze pad at tip to absorb blood while syringe plunger slowly pushed out the air and approximately 3 drops of blood.		
- Tore open the foiled cartridge pouch and removed the cartridge by holding the sides and placed it on a flat surface.		
- Held the syringe tip directly over sample well and carefully pushed the blood into the cartridge until the blood reached the arrow, and there was still blood remaining in the well but not overflowing.		
4. Moved the tab over the well from left to right using one finger; did not press on the beige circle area directly over the well; pushed down on the tab until it snapped into place.		
5. Used the grooved area to the left of the well or the sides of the cartridge to insert it slowly into the analyzer.		
- The handheld first displayed "Identifying Cartridge" and then a time-to-result bar.		
- ***Did not* remove cartridge until the "Cartridge Locked" message was removed and results were displayed on screen.**		
6. Reviewed results		
- After 2 to 3 minutes, the results appeared on the screen. The "n Page" command on bottom of the screen indicated more results would appear on a second screen. Pressed the print button to send the results to the printer by wireless transmission or by the docking device USB connection.		
- The handheld showed the numerical values and units with the results. It also showed bar graphs with tic marks for reference ranges.		
*Accurate Results _____ **Instructor Confirmation** _____		

Follow-up: Postanalytical Phase	Scores	
	S	U
*G. Proper documentation		
1. On control log: _____ yes _____ no		
2. On patient log: _____ yes _____ no		
3. Documented on patient chart (see below).		
4. Identified "critical values" and took appropriate steps to notify physician.		
*See table of test ranges below.		
H. Proper disposal and disinfection		
1. Disposed of all sharps in biohazard sharps containers.		
2. Disposed of all other regulated medical waste in biohazard bags.		
3. Disinfected test area and instruments according to OSHA guidelines.		
4. Sanitized hands after removing gloves.		
Total Points per Column		

Test	Test Symbol	Units	Reportable Range	Reference Range	Results	Critical Low/High
Sodium	Na	mmol/L	100-180	138-146		
Potassium	K	mmol/L	2.0-9.0	3.5-4.9		
Chloride	Cl	mmol/L	65-140	98-109		
Total carbon dioxide	TCO_2	mmol/L	5-50	24-29		
Ionized calcium	iCa	mmol/L	0.25-2.50	1.12-1.32		
Glucose	Glu	mg/dL	20-700	70-105		
Urea nitrogen	BUN	mg/dL	3-140	8-26		
Creatinine	Crea	mg/dL	0.2-20.0	0.6-1.3		
Hematocrit	Hct	% PCV	10-75	38-51		
Hemoglobin*	Hb	g/dL	3.4-25.5	12-17		
Anion gap*	AnGap	mmol/L	10-99	10-20		

Patient Name: _____

Attach printed readout, or record results on the chart above.

Procedure 6.5: Occult Blood: ColoScreen III Method

Person evaluated _____ Date _____

Evaluated by _____ Score _____

Outcome goal	To perform FDA-approved, CLIA-waived fecal occult blood test following the most current OSHA safety guidelines and applying the correct quality control
Conditions	Supplies needed: - Three specimen slides - Three wooden applicators - Hydrogen peroxide developer - Personal protective equipment
Standards	Required time: 5 minutes Performance time: _____ Total possible points = _____ Points earned = _____

Evaluation Rubric Codes:
S = Satisfactory, meets standard   **U** = Unsatisfactory, fails to meet standard

NOTE: Steps marked with an asterisk (*) are critical to achieve required competency.

Preparation: Preanalytical Phase	Scores	
	S	U
A. Test information		
- Kit or instrument method: **ColoScreen III**		
- Manufacturer: **SmithKline Diagnostics**		
- Proper storage (e.g., temperature, light): **room temperature**		
- Expiration date: _____		
- Lot # on kit: _____		
- Package insert or test flow chart available: _____ yes _____ no		
B. Instructed patient on the following dietary preparations:		
1. Two days before the test and during testing time, the patient should eat a high-fiber diet with any of the following:		
- Well-cooked poultry and fish		
- Cooked fruits and vegetables		
Bran cereals		
- Raw lettuce, carrots, and celery		
- Moderate amounts of peanuts and popcorn		
2. The patient should avoid ingesting the following substances, which interfere with the test results:		
- Red and partially cooked meats		
- Turnips, cauliflower, broccoli, parsnips, and melons (especially cantaloupe)		
- Alcohol, aspirin, and vitamin C		

	Scores	
C. Instructed the patient on how to use the slides, applicators, and the take-home instructions as follows:		
- After a bowel movement, use the wooden applicator to collect a small sample of feces, and spread a thin layer in box A of the slide.		
- Using the same applicator, collect a second sample from a different part of the feces, and spread it in box B.		
- Discard the wooden applicator, reseal the cover of the slide, and complete the information requested on the outside of the cover.		
- Repeat above steps with the remaining applicators for the next two bowel movements and two remaining slides.		

Procedure: Analytical Phase	Scores	
	S	U
D. Personal protective equipment: gloves when testing the slides		
E. Performed occult blood test as follows:		
- Confirmed all necessary information was written on slide covers.		
- Applied gloves and observed Universal Precautions.		
- Opened the back sides of all three slides and placed 2 drops of developer on each specimen.		
- Observed slide for 30 seconds to 2 minutes and checked to see if a blue reaction occurred, indicating a positive result.		
F. Performed monitor test (internal control)		
- Placed 1 or 2 drops between the monitor boxes and observed for 30 seconds to 2 minutes before reading the results.		
- Confirmed the positive control turned blue and the negative control did not.		
*Accurate Results _____ Instructor Confirmation _____		

Follow-up: Postanalytical Phase	Scores	
	S	U
G. Proper documentation		
1. On control/patient log: _____ yes _____ no		
2. Documented on patient chart (see following page).		
3. Identified critical values and took appropriate steps to notify physician.		
- Expected values for occult blood: negative		
H. Proper disposal and disinfection		
1. Disposed of all regulated medical waste in biohazard bags.		
2. Disinfected test area and instruments according to OSHA guidelines.		
3. Sanitized hands after removing gloves.		
Total Points per Column		

Patient Name: _____

Patient Chart Entry: (Include when, what, how, why, any additional information, and the signature of the person charting.)

_____

_____

_____

Procedure 6.6: Occult Blood: ColoCARE Method

Person evaluated _____   Date _____

Evaluated by _____   Score _____

Outcome goal	To perform FDA-approved, CLIA-waived fecal occult blood test at home following the most current OSHA safety guidelines and applying the correct quality control
Conditions	Supplies needed: - Patient receives foil packet containing three test pads and a reply card, along with an instruction sheet.

Evaluation Rubric Codes:
S = Satisfactory, meets standard   **U** = Unsatisfactory, fails to meet standard

NOTE: Steps marked with an asterisk (*) are critical to achieve required competency.

Preparation: Preanalytical Phase	Scores	
	S	U
A. Test information		
- Kit or instrument method: **ColoCARE**		
- Manufacturer: **Helena Laboratories**		
- Proper storage (e.g., temperature, light): **room temperature**		
- Expiration date: _____		
- Lot # on kit: _____		
- Package insert or test flow chart available: _____ yes _____ no		
B. Instructed patient on the following dietary preparations:		
1. Two days before the test and during testing time, the patient should eat a high-fiber diet with any of the following:		
- Well-cooked poultry and fish		
- Cooked fruits and vegetables		
- Bran cereals		
- Raw lettuce, carrots, and celery		
- Moderate amounts of peanuts and popcorn		
2. The patient should also avoid ingesting the following substances, which interfere with the test results:		
- Red and partially cooked meats		
- Turnips, cauliflower, broccoli, parsnips, and melons (especially cantaloupe)		
- Alcohol, aspirin, and vitamin C		
C. Instructed the patient on how to use the three test pads in the foil packet, the reply card, and the take-home testing instructions as follows:		

D. At Home Procedure Performed by Patient: Analytical Phase		
1. After a bowel movement, *do not flush or put toilet paper in the toilet.* **Perform the following steps within 5 minutes after bowel movement.**		
2. Open foil pouch by tearing along the dotted line at the bottom of the pouch, being careful not to tear the pad inside, and remove one ColoCARE pad from the pouch. Tape the pouch closed to protect the remaining pads from light and moisture.		
3. Hold the ColoCARE pad with the printed side up. Carefully release the pad, allowing it to float on the water in the center of the toilet bowl.		
4. Observe the ColoCARE pad for 30 seconds, and note any blue or green appearance on the pad below for possible negative and positive results.		
5. After testing the first bowel movement, mark the diagram on the reply card (Fig. D) labeled "First Bowel Movement" with an **"X" in each area of the pad that turned a blue or green color.** The areas include the large TEST AREA and the two smaller areas at the bottom of the pad (the positive and negative control areas). After recording the results on the reply card, flush the floating test pad down the toilet.		
6. Repeat step 5 for the next two consecutive bowel movements, and mark the second and third diagrams on the reply card according to the same instructions.		
7. Fill out all the information required on the reply card, and either mail it to the office or bring the card back to the office for interpretation.		
*Accurate Results _____ Instructor Confirmation _____		

	Scores	
Follow-up: Postanalytical Phase	S	U
E. Checked patient's returned report and confirmed the small internal control boxes had turned blue or green in the positive box and the patient wrote an "X" in the box and the negative control did not turn blue or green and had no "X" in the box.		
*F. Proper documentation		
1. On control/patient log: _____ yes _____ no		
2. Documented on patient chart.		
3. Identified critical values and took appropriate steps to notify physician.		
- Expected values for occult blood: negative (no "X's" in large box)		
G. Proper disposal and disinfection		
1. Disposed of all regulated medical waste in biohazard bags.		
2. Disinfected test area and instruments according to OSHA guidelines.		
3. Sanitized hands after removing gloves.		
Total Points per Column		

Patient Name: _____

Patient Chart Entry: (Include when, what, how, why, any additional information, and the signature of the person charting.)

_____

_____

_____

Procedure 6.7: Occult Blood: iFOB Method

Person evaluated _____   Date _____

Evaluated by _____   Score _____

Outcome goal	To perform FDA-approved, CLIA-waived fecal occult blood test using the most current OSHA safety guidelines and applying the correct quality control
Conditions	Supplies needed: **Patient supplies for collecting fecal specimen at home:** a. step-by-step illustrated instruction sheet; b. specimen collection paper to place across toilet seat; c. specimen collection tube with internal sampling probe to pierce the specimen; d. plastic biohazard bag and mailer to send specimen to the laboratory or office. **In-office testing cassette**: foil-wrapped testing cassette
Evaluation Rubric Codes: **S** = Satisfactory, meets standard **U** = Unsatisfactory, fails to meet standard	
NOTE: Steps marked with an asterisk (*) are critical to achieve required competency.	

A. Preparation: Preanalytical Phase	Scores	
	S	**U**
1. Test information		
- Kit or instrument method: **iFOB**		
- Manufacturer: **QuickVue by Quidel**		
- Proper storage (e.g., temperature, light): **room temperature**		
- Expiration date:		
- Lot # on kit:		
- Package insert or test flow chart available: yes no		
2. Instructed patient on the following dietary preparations:		
The QuickVue iFOB test is specific to human hemoglobin, and the patient does not need to follow the food restrictions of other fecal occult test methods. However, patients with the following conditions should not be considered for testing because these conditions may interfere with test results:		
- Menstrual bleeding		
- Bleeding hemorrhoids		
- Constipation bleeding		
- Urinary bleeding		
Patients with the above conditions may be considered for testing after bleeding ceases.		
- Alcohol and certain medications such as aspirin, indomethacin, reserpine, phenylbutazone, corticosteroids, and nonsteroidal antiinflammatory drugs may also cause gastrointestinal irritation and subsequent bleeding in some patients.		
3. Enter the patient identification information on the collection tube label.		

	Scores	

4. At home collection performed by patient:

    a. When collecting specimens, the patient should follow the take-home instructions as follows:

       - Do not collect specimen if bleeding is present from hemorrhoids, constipation, urination, or menstruation.

       - Urinate before positioning collection paper (or a paper plate).

       - Do not urinate on fecal specimen or collection paper.

       - Position paper on rear half of toilet seat and press the tape down on each side.

       - Deposit fecal specimen on the collection paper.

    b. Unscrew the dark blue Sampler probe from the collection tube that contains a liquid buffer solution.

       - Using the probe, pierce the specimen in at least five different sites.

       - Insert the sampler back into the collection tube, firmly tighten, and shake the tube well.

       - Flush remaining specimen and collection paper.

    c. Make sure patient ID line on the tube has the proper name on the label. Then insert the collection tube that has the well-mixed specimen and solution into:

       - absorbent sleeve,

       - then plastic specimen pouch,

       - then into the cardboard mailer.

       - Mail or bring the specimen to the medical office or laboratory.

B. Procedure: Analytical Phase Performed in the Office	Scores	
	S	U

Test performed in office.

1. Apply gloves and observe Universal Precautions. Confirm that all necessary information was written on the collection tube.

2. Shake tube well and unscrew pale blue cap.

3. Cover the exposed tip with the absorbent sleeve or gauze, and snap the tip away.

4. Squeeze 6 drops into the test well.

5. Read results as positive or negative or invalid after 5 to 10 minutes based on the following criteria:

    - Positive result: A pink line appears next to the letter "T" and next to the letter "C."

    - Negative result: Only one pink line forms next to the letter "C."

6. Invalid test: If there is no pink line next to the letter "C," the test results are invalid and should not be reported.

*Accurate Results _____ Instructor Confirmation _____

C. Follow-up: Postanalytical Phase	Scores	
	S	U

Proper documentation

1. On control/patient log: _____ yes _____ no

2. Documented on patient chart (see following page)

3. Identified critical values and took appropriate steps to notify physician

    - Expected values for occult blood: negative

Proper disposal and disinfection		
1. Disposed of all regulated medical waste in biohazard bags		
2. Disinfected test area and instruments according to OSHA guidelines		
3. Sanitized hands after removing gloves		
Total Points per Column		

Patient Name: _____

Patient Chart Entry: (Include when, what, how, why, any additional information, and the signature of the person charting.)

_____

_____

_____

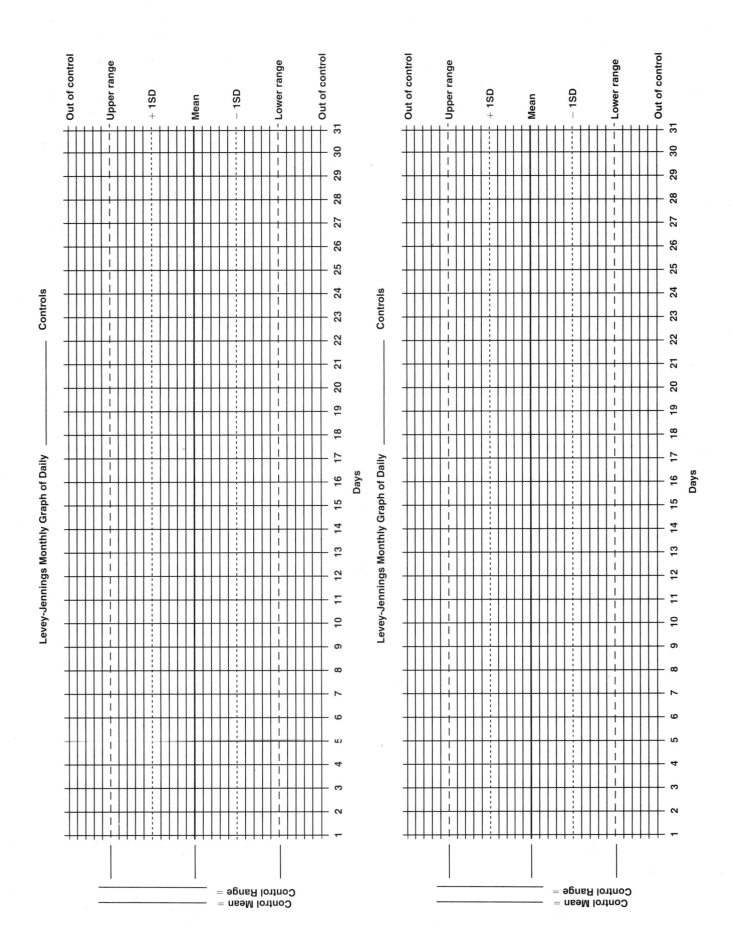

7 Immunology

VOCABULARY REVIEW

Match each definition with the correct term.

_____ 1. B-lymphocytic cell response to antigens resulting in the production of specific antibodies to destroy a foreign invader; also called antibody-mediated immunity

_____ 2. Cells capable of engulfing and ingesting microorganisms and cellular debris

_____ 3. Compound released by injured cells that causes dilation of blood vessels

_____ 4. Immunoglobulins produced specifically to destroy foreign invaders

_____ 5. Long-term protection against future infections resulting from the production of antibodies formed naturally during an infection or artificially by vaccination

_____ 6. Nonpathogenic microorganisms that normally inhabit the skin and mucous membranes

_____ 7. Overall reaction of the body to tissue injury or invasion by an infectious agent; characterized by redness, heat, swelling, and pain

_____ 8. Process of engulfing and digesting microorganisms and cellular debris

_____ 9. Proteins secreted by infected cells to prevent further replication and spread of an infection into neighboring cells

_____ 10. Proteins that stimulate phagocytosis and inflammation and are capable of destroying bacteria

_____ 11. Short-term acquired immunity created by antibodies received naturally through the placenta (or the colostrum to an infant) or artificially by injection

_____ 12. Special type of lymphocytes that attack and destroy infected cells and cancer cells in a nonspecific way

_____ 13. Substances that are perceived as foreign to the body and elicit an antibody response

_____ 14. T-lymphocytic cell response to antigens

_____ 15. Thin sheets of tissue that line the internal cavities and canals of the body and serve as a barrier against the entry of pathogens

_____ 16. Destructive tissue diseases caused by antibody/self-antigen reactions

A. active immunity
B. autoimmune diseases
C. antibodies
D. antigens
E. cell-mediated immunity
F. complement proteins
G. histamine
H. humoral immunity
I. inflammation
J. interferons
K. mucous membrane
L. natural killer cells
M. normal flora
N. passive immunity
O. phagocytes
P. phagocytosis

Match the B and T lymphocytes with their functions.

_____ 17. Antigen-activated B lymphocytes that remember an identified antigen for future encounters

_____ 18. Antigen-activated lymphocytes that attack foreign antigens directly and destroy cells that bear the antigens; also called cytotoxic cells

_____ 19. Antigen-activated lymphocytes that inhibit T and B cells after enough cells have been activated

_____ 20. Antigen-activated lymphocytes that stimulate other T cells and help B cells produce antibodies

_____ 21. Antigen-activated T lymphocytes that remember an antigen for future encounters

_____ 22. B lymphocytes that produce the antibodies that travel through the blood specifically targeting and reacting with antigens

A. killer T cells
B. suppressor T cells (regulatory T cells)
C. plasma cells
D. helper T cells (T_H4 or CD4)
E. memory B cells
F. memory T cells

Match the CLIA-WAIVED immunology testing and disease terms with their correct definitions.

_____ 23. Antibody that appears during an Epstein-Barr viral infection (mononucleosis) that has an unusual affinity to heterophile antigens on sheep red cells

_____ 24. Branch of laboratory medicine that performs antibody/antigen testing with serum

_____ 25. Clumping together of blood cells or latex beads caused by antibodies adhering to their antigens

_____ 26. A hemolytic anemia in newborns resulting from maternal–fetal blood group incompatibility

_____ 27. Testing in a laboratory apparatus

_____ 28. Pertaining to a visual color change that appears when an enzyme-linked antibody/antigen reaction occurs

_____ 29. Pertaining to the attachment of an antigen or antibody to a solid surface such as latex beads, wells in plastic dishes, or plastic cartridges

_____ 30. Process of injecting harmless or killed microorganisms into the body to induce immunity against a potential pathogen; also called immunization

_____ 31. Raised induration

_____ 32. Substances within the body that induce the production of antibodies that attack an individual's own body tissues; also called autoantigens

_____ 33. A quantitative test that measures the amount of antibody that reacts with a specific antigen

_____ 34. Testing within a host or living organism

A. agglutination
B. chromatographic assay
C. erythroblastosis fetalis
D. heterophile antibody
E. immunosorbent
F. in vitro
G. in vivo
H. self-antigens
I. serology
J. titer
K. vaccination
L. wheal

35. When a pathogen is invading the body, list two examples of protection for each line of defense:

    First line of external defenses: _____

    Second line of internal, nonspecific defenses: _____

    _____

    Third line of internal, specific defenses: _____

    _____

36. List two white cells that are phagocytic.

    _____

37. Give an example of a normal flora organism found in the female vagina, and describe how it prevents the invasion of pathogens.

    _____

    _____

38. List the four clinical signs of inflammation.

    _____

39. Describe antigens.

    _____

    _____

40. Which lymphocytic cells are associated with cell-mediated immunity?

    _____

41. What is another name for antibodies? (Hint: They are a subcategory of the globulin proteins.)

    _____

42. Name the five types of antibodies by their immunoglobulin identification (hint: they all start with Ig).

    _____

43. Refer to Fig. 7.4, *A* and *B*, in the textbook and give examples of natural and artificial active immunity and natural and artificial passive immunity.

    _____

    _____

44. The pregnancy test determines the presence of what antigenic substance?

   _____

   _____

45. Fill in the blanks for the following medical information regarding infectious mononucleosis:

   Causative agent: _____

   Clinical symptoms: _____

   Hematology findings: _____

   Immunology findings: _____

46. Label the QuickVue+ infectious mononucleosis supplies (see Procedure 7.2 in the textbook).

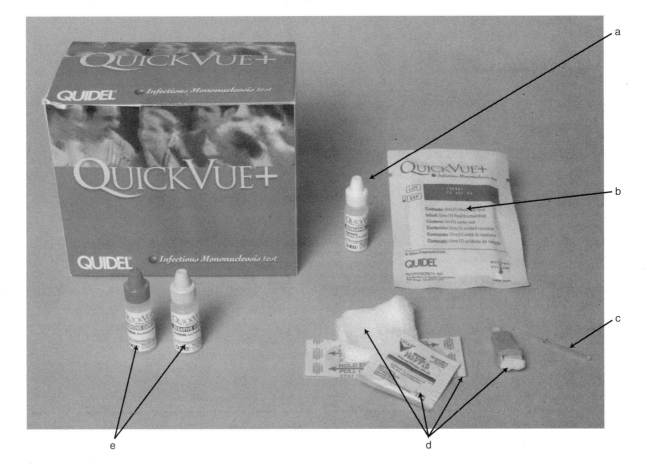

47. Describe the relationship between *Helicobacter pylori* and ulcers.

_____

_____

48. Indicate whether the following statements about HIV are TRUE or FALSE.

_____ a. HIV is now a curable disease.

_____ b. ARV (antiretroviral) is a medication that destroys HIV.

_____ c. Self-testing for HIV is now available.

_____ d. It is possible to receive a false-positive or a false-negative HIV test result.

49. Label the HIV supplies needed to perform the Uni-Gold Recombigen HIV blood test (see Procedure 7.4 figure A in the textbook).

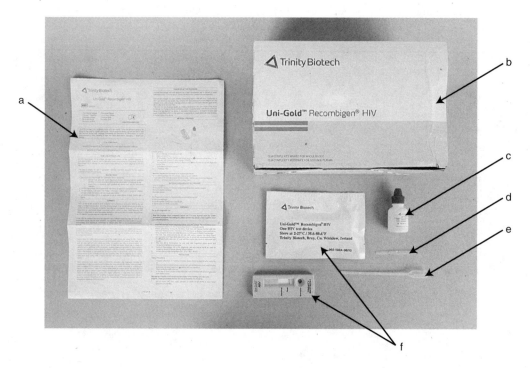

50. Based on the test results illustrated in the following chart, interpret the results for each test as **positive, negative,** or **invalid** based on the interpretation directions found in the textbook referenced figures.

	Test	Figure in Textbook	Interpreted Result
A.		**ICON hCG, Fig. 7.5**	
B.		**hCG Procedure 7.1, *B***	
C.		**Infectious Mononucleosis Procedure 7.2, *D***	

	Test	Figure in Textbook	Interpreted Result
D.		**HIV Blood Test Procedure 7.4, Fig. H, last figure on the right**	
E.		**HIV Blood Test Procedure 7.4, Fig. G, on the right (b)**	
F.		**HIV Blood Test Procedure 7.4, Fig. H, first figure on the left**	
G.		**HIV Blood Test Procedure 7.4, Fig. G, on the left (a)**	

ADVANCED CONCEPTS

51. Define agglutination.

_____

_____

52. Define immunohematology, and give three reasons why testing is done in this area.

_____

_____

53. Give the antigens and antibodies found in type AB blood. (See Table 7.2.)

_____

54. Would a woman with D antigen on her red blood cells be considered Rh positive or Rh negative? _____

    Would she be at risk for hemolytic disease of the newborn? _____

55. When the body is exposed to the following pathogens, it produces specific antibodies that can be measured in the plasma or serum. Refer to Table 7.3 in the textbook, identify the following pathogenic diseases, and indicate whether the pathogen is a bacterium or virus.

Pathogen	Disease	Bacterium or Virus
RSV		
Rubella		
Chlamydia		
Varicella zoster		
B. burgdorferi		

56. List three cancers that can be detected by immunologic testing (see Table 7.3 in the textbook). HINT: Look for "cancer" in "OTHER ANTIGENIC SUBSTANCES"

_____

_____

Procedure 7.1: SureStep Pregnancy Test Procedure

Person evaluated _____ Date _____

Evaluated by _____ Score/Grade _____

Outcome goal	To perform FDA-approved CLIA-waived urine pregnancy test following the most current OSHA safety guidelines and applying the correct quality control

Conditions	Supplies needed:
	- SureStep test kit containing:
	  - Individually wrapped test devices
	  - Disposal dropper pipettes
	  - Instruction insert
	- Other materials needed:
	  - Urine collection container
	  - Timer
	  - Liquid positive and negative controls for human chorionic gonadotropin (hCG)

Standards	Required time: 5 minutes Performance time: _____ Total possible points = _____ Points earned = _____

Evaluation Rubric Codes:
S = Satisfactory, meets standard   **U** = Unsatisfactory, fails to meet standard

NOTE: Steps marked with an asterisk (*) are critical to achieve required competency.

SureStep Pregnancy Test	Scores	
Preparation: Preanalytical Phase	S	U
A. Test information		
- Kit method: **SureStep**		
- Manufacturer: **Applied Biotech, Inc.**		
- Proper storage (e.g., temperature, light): **refrigerator or room temperature**		
- Lot # of kit: _____		
- Expiration date: _____		
- Package insert or test flow chart available: _____ yes _____ no		
B. Personal protective equipment: **gloves, gown, biohazard container**		
C. Specimen information: **clear urine specimen (centrifuge if cloudy)**		
- Type of specimen: **Preferably first morning urine specimen. Urine can be stored in refrigerator for 72 hours but must be tested at room temperature.**		
- Appropriate container: **clean, dry plastic or glass container**		
Procedure for SureStep hCG: Analytical Phase	Scores	
	S	U
D. Performed/observed qualitative quality control		
- External liquid controls: positive negative		
- Internal control: **Colored band appears in the control region (C).**		

	S	U
E. Performed patient test		
1. Sanitized hands and applied gloves.		
2. Removed test device from its protective pouch and labeled with patient identification.		
- Brought to room temperature before opening to avoid condensation.		
3. Drew up urine sample to the line marked on the pipette provided in kit.		
- Approximately 0.2 mL		
- Used separate pipettes and devices for each specimen and control		
4. Dispensed entire contents into the sample well.		
5. Waited for pink-colored bands to appear.		
- High concentrations of hCG can be observed in 40 seconds.		
- Low concentrations may need 4 minutes for the reaction time.		
- Did not interpret results after 10 minutes.		
6. At 5 minutes, read and recorded the results (circled result).		
- Positive = Two distinct pink bands appear, one in the patient test region (T) and one in the control region (C).		
- Negative = Only one pink band appears in the control region (C); no apparent pink band appears in the patient test region (T).		
- Invalid = a total absence of pink bands in control region; test must be repeated with a new device. If problem persisted, called for assistance.		

*Accurate Results _____ Instructor Confirmation _____

Follow-up: Postanalytical Phase	Scores	
	S	U
*F. Proper documentation		
1. On control/patient log: _____ yes _____ no		
2. Documented on patient chart (see below).		
3. Identified critical values and took appropriate steps to notify physician.		
- Expected values for analyte: negative for pregnancy		
G. Proper disposal and disinfection		
1. Disposed of all sharps in biohazard sharps containers.		
2. Disposed of all other regulated medical waste in biohazard bags.		
3. Disinfected test area and instruments according to OSHA guidelines.		
Total Points per Column		

Patient Name: _____

Patient Chart Entry: (Include when, what, how, why, any additional information, and the signature of the person charting.)

_____

_____

_____

Procedure 7.2: QuickVue+ Mononucleosis Test Procedure

Person evaluated _____ Date _____

Evaluated by _____ Score/Grade _____

Outcome goal	To perform FDA-approved CLIA-waived infectious mononucleosis test following the most current OSHA safety guidelines and applying the correct quality control

Conditions	Supplies needed:
	- QuickVue test kit containing:
	  - Developer
	  - Individually wrapped reaction units
	  - Capillary tubes for capillary blood and pipettes for venous blood
	  - Positive and negative liquid controls
	  - Instruction insert and pictorial flow chart
	- Other materials needed:
	  - Capillary puncture supplies (lancet, alcohol, gauze, bandage), or whole blood venipuncture specimen
	  - Timer
	  - Personal protective equipment

Standards	Required time: 10 minutes Performance time: _____ Total possible points = _____ Points earned = _____

Evaluation Rubric Codes:
S = Satisfactory, meets standard   **U** = Unsatisfactory, fails to meet standard

NOTE: Steps marked with an asterisk (*) are critical to achieve required competency.

Preparation for Mononucleosis Test: Preanalytical Phase	Scores	
	S	**U**
A. Test information		
- Kit method: **QuickVue1 Mononucleosis Test**		
- Manufacturer: **Quidel**		
- Proper storage (e.g., temperature, light): **room temperature**		
- Lot # of kit: _____		
- Expiration date: _____		
- Package insert or test flow chart available: _____ yes _____ no		
B. Personal protective equipment: **gloves, gown, biohazard container**		
C. Specimen information		
- Use the capillary transfer tube provided in the kit to obtain capillary blood or the larger transfer pipette in the kit to obtain the venipuncture whole blood and the liquid controls.		
Procedure for Mononucleosis: Analytical Phase	**S**	**U**
D. Performed/observed qualitative quality control		
- External liquid controls: positive _____ negative _____		
- Internal control: **The color blue fills the "read result" window.**		

157

	S	U
E. Performed patient test		
1. Dispensed all the blood from the capillary tube into the "add" well or transferred a large drop from the venous whole blood specimen with the pipette.		
2. Added 5 drops of developer to the "add" well.		
- Held bottle vertical and allowed drops to fall freely.		
3. Read results at 5 minutes.		
- "Test complete" line must be visible by 10 minutes.		
4. Interpretation of results (circled result):		
- Positive = Any shade of a blue vertical line forms a positive (+) sign in the "read result" window along with the blue "test complete" line. Even a faint blue vertical line should be reported as a positive result.		
- Negative = No blue vertical line appears in the "read result" window along with the blue "test complete" line.		
- Invalid = After 10 minutes, no signal is observed in the "test complete" window, or the color blue fills the "read result" window. If either occurs, the test must be repeated with a new reaction unit. If the problem continues, contact technical support.		
*Accurate Results _____ **Instructor Confirmation** _____	*	

Follow-up: Postanalytical Phase	Scores	
	S	U
F. Proper documentation		
1. On control/patient log: _____ yes _____ no		
2. Documented on patient chart (see below).		
3. Identified critical values and took appropriate steps to notify physician.		
- Expected values for analyte: negative for mononucleosis		
G. Proper disposal and disinfection		
1. Disposed of all sharps in biohazard sharps containers.		
2. Disposed of all other regulated medical waste in biohazard bags.		
3. Disinfected test area and instruments according to OSHA guidelines.		
4. Sanitized hands after removing gloves.		
Total Points per Column		

Patient Name: _____

Patient Chart Entry: (Include when, what, how, why, any additional information, and the signature of the person charting.)

_____

_____

_____

Procedure 7.3: QuickVue *Helicobacter pylori* gII Test (CLIA-Waived) Procedure

Person evaluated _____   Date _____

Evaluated by _____   Score/Grade _____

Outcome goal	To perform a CLIA-waived *H. pylori* test following the most current OSHA safety guidelines and applying the correct quality controls

Conditions	Supplies needed:
	- QuickVue *H. pylori* test kit containing:
	  - Foil-wrapped test cassettes
	  - Plastic capillary tubes for finger stick blood
	  - Disposable droppers for venous blood
	  - Liquid controls: positive and negative external controls
	  - Direction insert and procedure card
	- Other materials needed:
	  - Capillary puncture supplies (lancet, alcohol, gauze, bandage), or whole blood venipuncture specimen
	  - Timer
	  - Personal protective equipment

Standards	Required time: 10 minutes Performance time: _____ Total possible points = _____ Points earned = _____

Evaluation Rubric Codes:
S = Satisfactory, meets standard   **U** = Unsatisfactory, fails to meet standard

NOTE: Steps marked with an asterisk (*) are critical to achieve required competency.

Preparation for *H. pylori* Test: Preanalytical Phase	Scores	
	S	U
A. Test information		
- Kit method: **QuickVue *H. pylori* gII test**		
- Manufacturer: **Quidel**		
- Proper storage of kit: **room temperature**		
- Lot # of kit: _____		
- Expiration date: _____		
- Package insert or test flow chart available: _____ yes _____ no		
B. Personal protective equipment: **gloves, gown, biohazard container**		
C. Specimen information		
- Use the capillary tube provided in the kit to obtain capillary blood or the larger disposable dropper in the kit to obtain the venipuncture whole blood specimen and the liquid controls.		
Procedure for *H. pylori* Test: Analytical Phase	S	U
D. Performed/observed qualitative quality control.		
- External liquid controls: positive _____ negative _____		
- Internal control: **a blue band of color near the letter "C"**		

E. Performed patient test		
1. Dispensed the blood into the sample well by one of the following methods:		
- Transferred 1 large drop from the venous anticoagulated whole blood specimen with the disposable dropper.		
- Dispensed all the finger stick blood from the capillary tube.		
- Added 2 hanging drops of whole blood directly from a finger stick into the round sample well on the test cassette.		
2. Read and recorded results at 5 minutes.		
- Did not move the test cassette until the assay was complete.		
- Some positive results may be seen earlier than 5 minutes.		
3. Interpretation of results (circle result).		
- Positive = a pink line next to the letter "T" and a blue line next to the letter "C."		
- Negative = only a blue line next to the letter "C."		
- Invalid = no blue line next to the letter "C"; the test must be repeated with a new cassette. If the problem continues, contact technical support.		

*Accurate Results Instructor Confirmation

	Scores	
Follow-up: Postanalytical	**S**	**U**
*F. Proper documentation		
1. On control/patient log: _____ yes _____ no		
2. Documented on patient chart (see below).		
3. Identified critical values and took appropriate steps to notify physician.		
- Expected values for analyte: negative for *H. pylori*		
G. Proper disposal and disinfection		
1. Disposed of all sharps in biohazard sharps containers.		
2. Disposed of all other regulated medical waste in biohazard bags.		
3. Disinfected test area and instruments according to OSHA guidelines.		
4. Sanitized hands after removing gloves.		
Total Points per Column		

Patient Name: _____

Patient Chart Entry: (Include when, what, how, why, any additional information, and the signature of the person charting.)

_____

_____

_____

Procedure 7.4: Uni-Gold Recombigen HIV Blood Test

Person evaluated _____ Date _____

Evaluated by _____ Score/Grade _____

Outcome goal	To perform FDA-approved CLIA-waived **Uni-Gold Recombigen HIV Blood Test** following the most current OSHA safety guidelines and applying the correct quality control

Conditions	Supplies needed:
	- Uni-Gold test kit containing:
	  - Package insert and patient information sheets
	  - Box with 20 test devices
	  - Wash solution
	  - Finger stick sample collection and transfer pipette
	  - Disposable pipette to use with venipuncture whole blood
	  - Foil pouch and its test device
	  - Positive and negative controls
	  - Timer
	  - Personal protective equipment

Standards	Required time: 10 to 15 minutes (depending on blood collection method) Performance time: _____ Total possible points = _____ Points earned = _____

Evaluation Rubric Codes:
S = Satisfactory, meets standard   **U** = Unsatisfactory, fails to meet standard

NOTE: Steps marked with an asterisk (*) are critical to achieve required competency.

Preparation for Uni-Gold Recombigen HIV Blood Test: Preanalytical Phase	Scores	
	S	**U**
A. Test information		
- Kit method: **Uni-Gold Recombigen HIV Blood Test**		
- Manufacturer: **Trinity Biotech**		
- Proper storage (e.g., temperature, light): **room temperature**		
- Lot # of kit: _____		
- Expiration date: _____		
- Package insert or test flow chart available: _____ yes _____ no		
B. Personal protective equipment: gloves, gown, face mask, biohazard containers		
C. Specimen information		
- Use the capillary transfer tube provided in the kit to obtain capillary blood or the larger transfer pipette in the kit to obtain the venipuncture whole blood and the liquid controls.		
Procedure for Uni-Gold Recombigen HIV Blood Test: Analytical Phase	**S**	**U**
D. Performed/observed qualitative quality control		
- External liquid controls: positive _____ negative _____		
- Internal control: **The red line next to "CONTROL"**		
E. Performed patient test		
1. Sanitized hands, and applied personal protective equipment.		
2. Documented that the information sheet has been given to the patient and that the patient has read it.		

3. Allow the unopened foil packet and wash solution to come to room temperature. PERFORM ONLY ONE TEST AT A TIME.		
4. Open kit and lay the testing device on a clean flat surface.		
5. Label the device with the appropriate patient information.		
6. Collect the sample via venipuncture using EDTA (lavender-topped tube) or heparin (green-topped tube). Or, alternatively, collect the sample from a finger stick using the appropriate provided transfer pipette until the blood reaches the mark. It is important to hold the pipette gently in a horizontal position and to allow the blood to fill to the mark on the pipette.		

7. Add 1 free-flowing drop of the venous whole blood to the sample port (using the proper disposable transfer pipette in the kit).
     Or, alternatively, immediately dispense all the blood in the capillary pipette from the finger stick into the sample port.
     Note: Both of the above procedures should be done with a barrier shield or a full face mask to protect the operator from possible blood exposure to the mucous membranes.		

8. Discard the pipette in biohazard waste.		
9. Hold the dropper bottle of wash solution above the sample port in a vertical position, and add 4 free-flowing drops of the wash solution to the sample port.		

10. Do not move the test cassette until the assay is complete. Read and record the results of the test after 10 minutes but not more than 12 minutes:
    a. **Negative result**: Only one red line forms next to "Control."
    b. **Positive result**: A pink/red line appears next to "Test" and next to "Control." Report as "Preliminary Positive."
    c. **Invalid results**: For a test to be valid, a pink/red control line must be present, and the sample port must show a full red color. Refer to Fig. H in Test Procedure 7.4 for the five possible invalid results. If any of these results appear, do not report the patient result. The test must be repeated with a new testing device.		

*Accurate Results _____ Instructor Confirmation _____

Follow-up: Postanalytical Phase	Scores	
	S	U
11. Discard all the test materials in the appropriate biohazard containers.		
12. Remove and discard gloves in the biohazard container, and sanitize the hands.		
13. Proper documentation		
▪ On control/patient log: _____ yes _____ no		
▪ Documented on patient chart (see below).		
▪ Identified critical values and took appropriate steps to notify physician.		
- Expected values for analyte: negative		
Total Points per Column		

Patient Name: _____

Patient Chart Entry: (Include when, what, how, why, any additional information, and the signature of the person charting.)

_____

_____

_____

Procedure 7.5: HIV OraQuick Test

Person evaluated _____ Date _____

Evaluated by _____ Score/Grade _____

Outcome goal	To perform FDA-approved CLIA-waived HIV OraQuick Test following the most current OSHA safety guidelines and applying the correct quality control

Conditions	**OraQuick HIV self-test kit contents:**
	- Box and its white plastic test kit containing the flip chart directions and the following displayed items located in the pull-out drawer:
	  - Required manufacturer's insert and pencil for writing start and finish times
	  - Plastic bag for disposal of the test supplies when finished
	  - Foil-wrapped test stick and test tube
	  - Two booklets titled "Please Read This Book First—HIV, Testing, and Me" and "What Your Results Mean to You!"
	Additional items (if performing the HIV OraQuick Test in the office):
	- Positive and negative external liquid controls
	- Personal protective equipment including gloves, face protection, gown, and OSHA disposal equipment

Standards	Required time: 30 to 50 minutes (based on setting up test and incubation time of 20 to 40 minutes) Performance time: _____ Total possible points = _____ Points earned = _____

Evaluation Rubric Codes:
S = Satisfactory, meets standard   **U** = Unsatisfactory, fails to meet standard

NOTE: Steps marked with an asterisk (*) are critical to achieve required competency.

Preparation for HIV OraQuick Test: Preanalytical Phase	Scores S	Scores U
A. Test information		
- Kit method: **HIV OraQuick Test**		
- Manufacturer: **OraQuick**		
- Proper storage (e.g., temperature, light): **room temperature**		
- Lot # of kit: _____		
- Expiration date: _____		
- Package insert or test flow chart available: _____ yes _____ no		
B. Personal protective equipment: gloves, gown, face mask, biohazard containers		
C. Patient preparation		
- Most people feel a little bit anxious when taking an HIV test. If patients feel very anxious about taking the self-test, they may want to wait until they are calmer or get tested by a physician at a local clinic.		
- It is important not to eat, drink, or use oral care products (e.g., mouthwash, toothpaste, or whitening strips) within 30 minutes before starting the test.		
- Remove dental products such as dentures or any other products that cover the gums.		
- Find a quiet, well-lit place where you can stay for at least 20 minutes.		
- You must follow the test directions carefully to get an accurate result.		
- Make sure you have a timer, watch, or something that can time 20 to 40 minutes.		

Procedure for HIV OraQuick Self-Test or In-Office Test: Analytical Phase	S	U
D. Performing the test.		
1. Sanitize the hands, and apply personal protective equipment.		
2. Ensure that the pretest booklet "Please Read This Book First" has been given to the patient and that the patient has read it.		
3. Open kit drawer and lay out all supplies.		
4. With the white plastic lid in the open position, proceed by following the directions and demonstrations on each of the numbered flip charts:		
Step 1: Open Test Tube—Find the packet labeled "Test Tube" and tear open the packet to remove the test tube.		
Step 2: Set Up—Be careful! There's liquid at the bottom of the tube. Hold the tube upright. Gently *pop* off the test tube's cap—do not twist. Put the test tube in the holder labeled "Test Tube Holder," located on the right side of the plastic lid that is opened and upright.		
Step 3: Open Test Stick—Locate the packet labeled "Test Stick." Tear open the packet and remove the test stick being careful not to touch the pad with your fingers.		
Step 4: Swipe Gums—(Make sure the timer is ready and set for 20 minutes, but do not start it yet.) Gently swipe the pad along the upper gums once and then the lower gums once. Make sure you swipe the pad between the gum and the lips from one side all the way to the other on both the upper and the lower gums.		
Step 5: Drop in and Start Timing—Put the test stick pad directly into the test tube located on the right side of the plastic lid and start the timer for 20 minutes. Note: The kit also provides a pencil and a place to write in the start time, the time after 20 minutes, and the time after 40 minutes.		
Step 6: Wait 20 minutes—The test kit provides a flap to cover the test area on the stick. The area will turn pink for a few minutes. That is normal. Do not read the results before 20 minutes (this may give a wrong result). Read the results between 20 and 40 minutes. After 40 minutes, the test will no longer be accurate. While waiting for the results, the patient should read the second booklet, "What Your Results Mean to You!"		
Step 7: Reading Your Results—Move the flap that covered the test area to see the results. Compare the test stick with the pictures on the flip chart. If the results do not look like the examples on the flip chart or there are no lines on the test stick, the test is not working. For questions, call toll-free 1-866-436-6527.		
NOTE: A positive result with this test does not mean the person tested is definitely infected with HIV, but rather that additional testing should be done in a medical setting. A negative result with this test does not mean that a person is definitely not infected with HIV, particularly when exposure may have been within the previous 3 months.		
Step 8: Dispose—Remove the test stick, put the cap on the test tube, and place all the contents in the disposal bag provided in the test kit and throw it away.		
For questions, call toll-free 1-866-436-6527		
*Accurate Results _____ Instructor Confirmation _____		

Follow-up: Postanalytical Phase	Scores	
	S	U
E. Proper documentation		
■ On control/patient log: _____ yes _____ no		
■ Documented on patient chart.		
■ Identified critical values and took appropriate steps to notify physician.		
- Expected values for analyte: negative		
Total Points per Column		

Patient Name: _____

Patient Chart Entry: (Include when, what, how, why, any additional information, and the signature of the person charting.)

_____

_____

_____

<u>**GENERIC ANALYTICAL TEST FORM (FOR KITS NOT COVERED IN THE TEXTBOOK OR WORKBOOK)**</u>

Qualitative Test: _____

Person evaluated _____ Date _____

Evaluated by _____ Score/Grade _____

Outcome goal	
Conditions	Supplies required:
Standards	Required time: _____
	Performance time: _____
	Total possible points = _____ Points earned = _____
Evaluation Rubric Codes: **S** = Satisfactory, meets standard **U** = Unsatisfactory, fails to meet standard	
NOTE: Steps marked with an asterisk (*) are critical to achieve required competency.	

Preparation: Preanalytical Phase	Scores	
	S	**U**
A. Test information		
- Kit method:		
- Manufacturer:		
- Proper storage (e.g., temperature, light):		
- Lot # of kit: _____		
- Expiration date: _____		
- Package insert or test flow chart available: _____ yes _____ no		
B. Personal protective equipment:		
C. Specimen information		

Procedure: Analytical Phase	Scores	
	S	**U**
D. Performed/observed qualitative quality control		
- External liquid controls: positive _____ negative _____		
- Internal control		
E. Performed patient test		
1.		
2.		
3.		
4.		
Positive = Negative = Invalid =		
*Accurate Results _____ Instructor Confirmation _____		

Follow-up: Postanalytical Phase	Scores	
	S	U
*F. Proper documentation		
1. On control/patient log: _____ yes _____ no		
2. Documented on patient chart (see below).		
3. Identified critical values and took appropriate steps to notify physician.		
- Expected values for analyte:		
G. Proper disposal and disinfection		
1. Disposed of all sharps in biohazard sharps containers.		
2. Disposed of all other regulated medical waste in biohazard bags.		
3. Disinfected test area and instruments according to OSHA guidelines.		
4. Sanitized hands after removing gloves.		
Total Points per Column		

Patient Name: _____

Patient Chart Entry: (Include when, what, how, why, any additional information, and the signature of the person charting.)

_____

_____

_____

8 Microbiology

VOCABULARY REVIEW

Match each definition with the correct term.

_____ 1. Rate at which illness occurs

_____ 2. Displaying the pink or red color of the counterstain used in Gram's method of staining microorganisms

_____ 3. Diffuse muscle pain

_____ 4. Pertaining to unicellular organisms that do not have a true nucleus with a nuclear membrane

_____ 5. Displaying the purple color of the primary stain used in Gram's method of staining microorganisms

_____ 6. Disease that occurs when pathogenic microorganisms invade the body and overcome its natural defense mechanisms

_____ 7. Coughing up sputum and mucus from the trachea and lungs

_____ 8. Component made of polysaccharides and peptides that gives rigidity to the bacterial cell wall

_____ 9. Feeling of weakness, distress, or discomfort

_____ 10. Requiring special nutrients in media for growth

_____ 11. Pertaining to organisms that possess a true nucleus with a nuclear membrane and organelles

_____ 12. Rate of deaths

_____ 13. Asexual reproduction in which the cell splits in half

_____ 14. Mucus expelled from the lungs

_____ 15. Identification of the antibiotic of choice to treat an infection

_____ 16. Containing pus

A. malaise
B. myalgia
C. expectoration
D. gram positive
E. fastidious
F. mortality
G. gram negative
H. infection
I. peptidoglycan
J. morbidity
K. eukaryotic
L. prokaryote
M. binary fission
N. sensitivity test
O. purulent
P. sputum

FUNDAMENTAL CONCEPTS

17. Give an example of an organism that is normal flora, and discuss what can occur if the organism is destroyed.

_____

_____

18. Using Table 8.1 in the textbook, list the three most recent health issues of concern from 2013 through 2016.

_____

_____

19. List four characteristics of bacteria.

_____

_____

20. Explain the difference between a yeast fungus and a mold fungus.

_____

_____

21. List the three general types of bacterial shapes, and give an example of each.

_____

_____

22. Match each bacterial shape or group with its name (see Fig. 8.1 in the textbook).

_____   A. Bacilli

_____   B. Spirilla

_____   C. Streptococci

_____   D. Staphylococci

_____   E. Diplococci

23. Describe the benefits that flagella, spores, and capsules give to organisms that possess these structures.

_____

_____

_____

24. List four ways that medical assistants can take precautions to prevent the spread of infection to others or to themselves.

_____

_____

25. When is the ideal time to collect a microbiology specimen?

_____

_____

26. Discuss the swab kit for the DNA probe transport system (see Fig. 8.7).

_____

_____

27. Describe the cell wall structures that cause some organisms to be gram positive or gram negative.

_____

_____

28. Give the color of gram-positive and gram-negative organisms after the decolorizer step has been applied

_____

_____

29. Label the supplies needed for Gram staining (see Procedure 8.2 in the textbook).

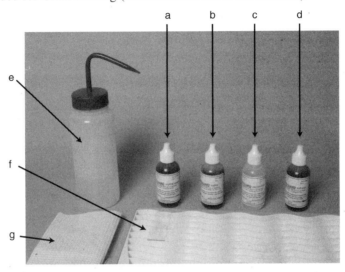

30. What is the causative agent for tuberculosis?

_____

_____

31. Describe the appearance and characteristics of *Trichomonas vaginalis.*

_____

_____

_____

32. Case study: On each blank, write **C** if the statement is correct and **I** if the statement is incorrect. If the step is incorrect, explain why in the space provided.
    A medical assistant is performing Gram staining of a specimen.

    _____ 1. The specimen is heat fixed to the slide.

_____

    _____ 2. Crystal violet is applied to the slide for 2 minutes and then rinsed with water.

_____

    _____ 3. Gram's iodine is applied for 1 minute, and both gram-positive and gram-negative organisms stain purple. Rinse with water.

_____

_____ 4. The decolorizer is applied until the purple has stopped running off the slide. This is the most critical step. Rinse with water.

_____ 5. Safranin is applied last for 1 minute and rinsed with water. Gram-positive organisms stain pink or red, and gram-negative organisms stain purple.

PROCEDURES: CLIA-WAIVED MICROBIOLOGY TESTS

33. Describe the appearance of alpha, beta, and gamma hemolysis on blood agar plates.

_____

_____

_____

34. State the causative agent (genus and species) of strep throat, and give the most common hemolytic reaction that this organism produces on blood agar plates.

_____

_____

_____

35. What antibiotic is in the disk that is used to identify *Streptococcus pyogenes*?

_____

36. Label the supplies needed to perform a group A *Streptococcus* test (see Procedure 8.5 in the textbook).

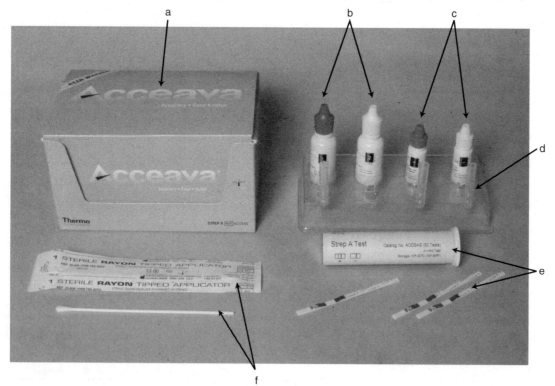

37. List three medical conditions associated with a strep infection.

_____

_____

_____

38. When discussing influenza, what is the difference between antigenic *drift* and *shift*?

_____

_____

_____

39. Describe how to obtain a nasal swab specimen when testing for influenza.

_____

_____

ADVANCED CONCEPTS

40. Give the oxygen requirements for aerobic and anaerobic organisms.

_____

_____

41. Name media requirements that most bacteria need for growth.

_____

_____

42. Give the advantages of using an incinerator instead of a Bunsen burner.

_____

_____

43. Describe or draw a picture of the differences between quadrant streaking and colony count streaking.

_____

_____

44. Explain a physician's reason for ordering a sensitivity test.

_____

_____

45. List three organisms that frequently cause urinary tract infections.

_____

_____

46. Case study: Refer to the text section "Pathogenic Organisms Seen Frequently in Physician Office Laboratories" and use Tables 8.4 through 8.9 in the textbook to complete the following information regarding common pathogenic bacteria:

Streptococcus pneumoniae

- Gram stain reaction: _____
- Disease: _____
- Transmission: _____
- Specimens: _____

Neisseria gonorrhoeae

- Gram stain reaction: _____
- Disease: _____
- Transmission: _____
- Specimens: _____

Chlamydia trachomatis

- Disease: _____
- Transmission: _____
- Specimens: _____

Enterobius vermicularis

- Transmission: _____
- Specimens or tests: _____

Urinary tract infections

- Organisms: _____
- Gram stain reaction: _____
- Transmission: _____
- Tests or specimen: _____

Food poisoning (most common cause in the United States)

- Organisms: _____
- Gram stain reaction: _____
- Transmission: _____
- Tests or specimen: _____

Procedure 8.1: Procedure for Collecting a Throat Specimen

Person evaluated _____   Date _____

Evaluated by _____   Score/Grade _____

Outcome goal	To perform throat specimen collection
Conditions	Supplies needed: - Sterile swabs and tongue depressor - Personal protective equipment
Standards	Required time: 10 minutes Performance time: _____ Total possible points = _____ Points earned = _____

Evaluation Rubric Codes:
S = Satisfactory, meets standard   **U** = Unsatisfactory, fails to meet standard

NOTE: Steps marked with an asterisk (*) are critical to achieve required competency.

Preparation	Scores	
	S	U
*1. Identified patient and placed in proper position.		
- Had patient state name.		
- Confirmed identification with patient.		
- Compared with requisition.		

Procedure	Scores	
	S	U
*2. Sanitized hands and put on gloves and face mask.		
*3. Aseptically removed the sterile Dacron swab (cotton swab may inhibit growth of bacteria) from the package, holding only the tip of the swab.		
*4. Had the patient sit with head back.		
*5. Used a sterile tongue depressor to hold down the tongue and had patient say "ahh."		
*6. Rotated the swab on the back of throat in a circular motion or figure-eight pattern.		
- Did not touch the teeth or back of the tongue because these areas have normal flora.		
- Two swabs can be used at the same time: one for a rapid strep test and one for a culture if needed.		
7. Inserted swab into appropriate container for testing.		

Follow-up	Scores	
	S	U
8. Determined if patient was feeling well before dismissing.		
*9. Completed proper documentation on patient chart (see below).		
*10. Proper disposal and disinfection.		
- Disinfected test area and instruments according to OSHA guidelines.		
- Disposed of regulated medical waste (e.g., gloves, tongue depressor) in biohazard bags.		
*11. Sanitized hands.		
Total Points per Column		

Patient Name: _____

Patient Chart Entry: (Include when, what, why, how, any additional information, and the signature of the person charting.)

_____

_____

_____

Procedure 8.2: Gram Stain Procedure

Person evaluated _____ Date _____

Evaluated by _____ Score/Grade _____

Outcome goal	Perform a Gram stain on a fixed smear on a slide
Conditions	Supplies needed: - Gloves, bibulous paper, water bottle or running water - Gram staining reagents: crystal violet, Gram's iodine, decolorizer, safranin - Staining rack
Standards	Required time: 15 minutes Performance time: _____ Total possible points = _____ Points earned = _____ Accuracy = final slide shows gram-positive and gram-negative bacteria

Evaluation Rubric Codes:
S = Satisfactory, meets standard   **U** = Unsatisfactory, fails to meet standard

NOTE: Steps marked with an asterisk (*) are critical to achieve required competency.

Preparation	Scores S	U
*1. Sanitized hands and applied gloves.		
*2. Fixed specimen to the slide (using heat or methanol).		
Procedure	**Scores** S	**U**
*3. Applied crystal violet to slide for 1 minute.		
*4. Rinsed slide with water.		
*5. Applied Gram's iodine to slide for 1 minute.		
*6. Rinsed slide with water.		
*7. Poured decolorizer over the tilted slide until no more purple ran off (about 3 to 5 seconds), and then immediately rinsed slide with water to stop the reaction.		
*8. Applied safranin stain for 1 minute.		
9. Rinsed slide with water.		
10. Blotted slide dry in absorbent bibulous paper.		
Follow-up	**Scores** S	**U**
*11. Proper disposal and disinfection.		
- Disinfected test area and instruments according to OSHA guidelines.		
- Disposed of regulated medical waste (e.g., gloves) in biohazard bags.		
- Sanitized hands.		
Totals Points per Column		

Patient Name: _____

Patient Chart Entry:

_____

_____

_____

Procedure 8.5: Acceava Strep A Test Procedure

Person evaluated _____ Date _____

Evaluated by _____ Score/Grade _____

Outcome goal	To perform FDA-approved, CLIA-waived rapid strep test following the most current OSHA safety guidelines and applying the correct quality control
Conditions	Supplies required: - Acceava rapid strep kit containing: - Reagent 1 and reagent 2 - Liquid controls, positive and negative - Soft plastic testing tubes - Test stick and its container - Sterile rayon swab taken from wrapper - Sterile tongue depressor - Gloves, face protection
Standards	Required time: 10 minutes Performance time: _____ Total possible points = _____ Points earned = _____

Evaluation Rubric Codes:
S = Satisfactory, meets standard   **U** = Unsatisfactory, fails to meet standard

NOTE: Steps marked with an asterisk (*) are critical to achieve required competency.

Preparation: Preanalytical Phase	Scores S	Scores U
A. Test information		
- Kit or instrument method: **Strep A Test**		
- Manufacturer: **Acceava**		
- Proper storage (e.g., temperature, light): **room temperature**		
- Lot # of kit: _____		
- Expiration date: _____		
- Package insert or test flow chart available: _____ yes _____ no		
B. Specimen information		
- Type of specimen: **throat swab using swab from kit (do not use cotton swabs)**		
C. Personal protective equipment: **gloves, face mask during throat swab, and biohazard container**		

Procedure: Analytical Phase	Scores S	Scores U
D. Performed/observed qualitative quality control		
- External liquid controls: positive _____ negative _____		
- Internal control: _____ (appears as a red line on test stick)		
E. Performed patient test		
1. Sanitized hands and applied gloves.		
2. Just before testing, added 3 drops of reagent 1 and 3 drops of reagent 2 into the test tube. The solution should turn light yellow.		

	Scores	
	S	**U**
3. Immediately put the throat swab into the extract solution.		
4. Vigorously mixed the solution by rotating the swab forcefully against the side of the tube at least 10 times. Best results are obtained when the specimen is vigorously extracted in the solution.		
5. Let stand for 1 minute, and then squeezed the swab with the sides of the tube as the swab was withdrawn; discarded the swab into a biohazard container.		
6. Removed a test stick from the container and recapped immediately; placed the absorbent end of the test stick into the extracted sample in the tube.		
7. At 5 minutes, read and recorded the results.		
- Positive = a blue line in test area and pink line in control area, indicating the internal control worked.		
- Negative = no blue line in the test area and a pink line in control area, indicating the internal control worked.		

*Accurate Results _____ **Instructor Confirmation** _____

Follow-up: Postanalytical Phase	Scores	
	S	**U**
*F. Proper documentation		
1. On control/patient log: _____ yes _____ no		
2. Documented on patient chart (see below).		
3. Identified critical values and took appropriate steps to notify physician.		
- Expected values for analyte: negative for strep		
G. Proper disposal and disinfection		
1. Disposed of all sharps in biohazard sharps containers.		
2. Disposed of all other regulated medical waste in biohazard bags.		
3. Disinfected test area and instruments according to OSHA guidelines.		
4. Sanitized hands after removing gloves.		
Totals Points per Column		

Patient Name: _____

Patient Chart Entry: (Include when, what, how, why, any additional information, and the signature of the person charting.)

_____

_____

_____

Procedure 8.6: OSOM Influenza A&B Test Procedure

Person evaluated _____ Date _____

Evaluated by _____ Score/Grade _____

Outcome goal	To perform FDA-approved CLIA-waived influenza test following the most current OSHA safety guidelines and applying the correct quality control
Conditions	Supplies required for the OSOM Influenza A&B Test: - Personal protective equipment (disposable gown, face mask, and gloves) - Foam swab provided in kit to collect nasal specimen - Plastic testing tube provided in kit - Extract solution provided in kit - Testing strip provided in kit - Control swabs for influenza A and B - Container of testing strips with diagram showing how to interpret results
Standards	Required time: 10 minutes Performance time: _____ Total possible points = _____ Points earned = _____
Evaluation Rubric Codes: **S** = Satisfactory, meets standard **U** = Unsatisfactory, fails to meet standard	
NOTE: Steps marked with an asterisk (*) are critical to achieve required competency.	

Preparation: Preanalytical Phase	Scores S	Scores U
A. Test information		
- Kit or instrument method: **OSOM A&B Influenza Test**		
- Manufacturer: **Genzyme**		
- Proper storage (e.g., temperature, light): **room temperature**		
- Lot # of kit: _____		
- Expiration date: _____		
- Package insert or test flow chart available: _____ yes _____ no		
B. Specimen information		
- Type of specimen: **nasal swab using swab from kit**		
- **Sanitize hands and apply gloves and face mask**		
- Insert the foam swab provided in the test kit into the patient's nostril displaying the most secretion. Using a gentle rotation, push the swab until resistance is met at the level of the turbinates (at least 1 inch into the nostril). Rotate the swab a few times against the nasal wall, and gently rock it back and forth. Hold swab in place for 5 seconds to ensure maximum absorbency.		
C. Personal protective equipment: gloves during testing		

Procedure: Analytical Phase	Scores S	Scores U
D. Performed/observed qualitative quality control		
- External swab controls: Positive A _____ Positive B _____		
Negative A _____ Negative B _____		
- Internal control appears as a blue line on test stick.		

		S	U
E. Performed patient test			
1. Sanitized hands and applied gloves.			
2. Placed the nasal swab into the plastic tube containing the designated amount of extraction buffer solution.			
3. Vigorously twisted the swab against the sides and bottom of the tube at least 10 times, which disrupted the virus particles and released the internal viral nucleoproteins into the solution.			
4. Extracted all the solution from the swab by squeezing the plastic tube against the swab while removing it from the tube and disposed of swab properly.			
5. Dipped the influenza test strip into the tube with the extraction buffer, making sure the arrows on the strip were pointing down.			
6. Allowed 10 minutes for migration of the solution across the test area and control area of the strip, which allowed the nucleoproteins from the virus to react with the reagents on the test strip, causing a color reaction.			
7. Read the results for the influenza A and B test.			
- Positive = Result showed a pink or purple line in the A or B test area and a pink line in the internal control area.			
- Negative = Result showed no color change in the A or B test area and a pink line in the internal control area.			

*Accurate Results _____   Instructor Confirmation _____

Follow-up: Postanalytical Phase	Scores	
	S	U
*F. Proper documentation		
1. On control/patient log: _____ yes _____ no		
2. Documented on patient chart (see below).		
3. Identified critical values and took appropriate steps to notify physician.		
- Expected values for analyte: negative for influenza A and B		
G. Proper disposal and disinfection		
1. Disposed of all sharps in biohazard sharps containers.		
2. Disposed of all other regulated medical waste in biohazard bags.		
3. Disinfected test area and instruments according to OSHA guidelines.		
4. Sanitized hands after removing gloves.		
Totals Counts per Column		

Patient Name: _____

Patient Chart Entry: (Include when, what, how, why, any additional information, and the signature of the person charting.)

_____

_____

_____

Procedure 8.7: Rapid Urine Culture Test

Person evaluated _____ Date _____

Evaluated by _____ Score/Grade _____

Outcome goal	To perform FDA-approved CLIA-moderate complexity **Rapid Urine Culture Test** following the most current OSHA safety guidelines and applying the correct quality control
Conditions	**Equipment and Supplies** - Clinical incubator - Uricult kit containing vial with agar-coated slide and reference chart - Gloves - Requisition
Standards	Required time: overnight incubation (18 to 24 hours) Performance time: _____ Total possible points = _____ Points earned = _____

Evaluation Rubric Codes:
S = Satisfactory, meets standard   **U** = Unsatisfactory, fails to meet standard

NOTE: Steps marked with an asterisk (*) are critical to achieve required competency.

Preparation: Preanalytical Phase	Scores	
	S	**U**
A. Test information		
- Kit or instrument method: **Uricult**		
- Manufacturer: **LifeSign**		
- Proper storage (e.g., **temperature**, light): **room temperature**		
- Lot # of kit: _____		
- Expiration date: _____		
- Package insert or test flow chart available: _____yes _____no		
B. Specimen information: Have the patient produce a freshly voided clean-catch midstream urine sample that has been in the bladder for a minimum of 4 to 6 hours in the appropriate container. Be sure to mix the urine sample before testing.		
C. Daily monitoring and logging of incubator temperature must be documented.		
D. Personal protective equipment: gloves and gown during testing		

Procedure: Analytical Phase	Scores	
	S	**U**
E. **Quality Control:** No quality control testing required. Visually inspect Uricult vials for contamination, excess moisture, and damage before use. Remove Certificate of Analysis from package insert and document.		
F. No standard proficiency survey is required, but the office must participate in a biannual assessment program.		
G. Perform the urine culture test.		
1. Unscrew the agar-coated slide from the vial being careful not to touch the agar.		
2. Completely immerse the slide into the urine making sure the agar on both sides of the slide is not immersed for more than several seconds. (Note: If the urine volume in the cup is too small to dip, the urine may be poured over the agar surfaces.)		

	Scores	
3. Place the urine-dipped specimen back into the vial and screw the cap on loosely. Label the vial with the patient's name, date, time, and your initials. Place in the incubator.		
4. Read results using reference chart supplied in kit after 18 to 24 hours of incubation (do not exceed 24 hours). Results are interpreted as follows:		
- *Normal:* Color that reads as <10,000 bacteria/mL of urine indicates the absence of infection.		
- *Borderline:* Color that reads 10,000 to 100,000 bacteria/mL of urine may indicate a chronic or relapsing infection; it is recommended that the test be repeated.		
- *Positive:* Color that reads >100,000 bacteria/mL of urine showing complete coverage of the agar surface with bacterial colonies.		
5. Replace the agar slide in the vial and discard in a biohazard bag. Disinfect test area and instruments according to OSHA guidelines.		

*Accurate Results _____   **Instructor Confirmation** _____

Follow-up: Postanalytical Phase	Scores	
	S	U
6. Remove the gloves, and sanitize your hands.		
*G. Proper Documentation		
1. On control/patient log: _____ yes _____ no		
2. Documented on patient chart (see below).		
3. Identified critical values and took appropriate steps to notify physician.		
- Expected values for analyte: negative for bacterial infection		
Totals Points per Column		

Patient Name: _____

Patient Chart Entry: (Include when, what, why, how, any additional information, and the signature of the person charting.)

_____

_____

_____

9 Toxicology

VOCABULARY REVIEW

Match each definition with the correct term.

_____ 1. Methadone and morphine

_____ 2. The transport of a drug through the body by the blood

_____ 3. A measurement that determines whether a substance is present or absent

_____ 4. An abnormal susceptibility to a drug or other agent that is peculiar to the individual

_____ 5. When a prescribed drug has entered the body and has released the active component

_____ 6. The level at which a drug becomes poisonous in the body

_____ 7. A precise measurement of the amount of a substance present in a specimen

_____ 8. The primary psychoactive compound in marijuana

_____ 9. The movement of a substance through the surface of the body into body fluids and tissues

_____ 10. An FDA-approved drug for treating opioid drug addiction

_____ 11. The movement of drugs through the body from the time of introduction to elimination

_____ 12. A substance produced by the metabolism (breaking down) of a drug in the body

A. idiosyncrasy
B. pharmacokinetics
C. opioids
D. toxicity
E. qualitative drug screening
F. absorption
G. liberation
H. quantitative
I. buprenorphine
J. distribution
K. cannabinoid
L. metabolite

FUNDAMENTAL CONCEPTS

13. List three reasons a specimen would be tested in a toxicology laboratory.

_____

_____

_____

14. List three toxicology responsibilities in the ambulatory care setting.

_____

_____

_____

15. Explain three ways an over-the-counter (OTC) drug can become toxic.

_____

_____

_____

16. Define what makes a drug of abuse.

_____

_____

17. When testing for a drug, urine is usually used for a(n) _____ result, and blood is used for a(n) _____ result.

18. Describe the *chain of custody* when processing a specimen for drug screening for the Department of Transportation (DOT).

_____

_____

19. Define MRO.

_____

_____

20. Explain the three results in the urine drug test illustration (Fig. D in Procedure 9.3).

COC _____

AMP _____

mAMP _____

21. Using Table 9.3, write the drug name that matches the following testing codes:

THC _____

COC _____

BUP _____

OPI _____

BAR _____

BZO _____

MTD _____

AMP _____

OXY _____

mAMP _____

22. Why is it important to monitor drug levels during drug therapy?

    _____

    _____

23. From Table 9.4, list the six drug categories that require therapeutic monitoring.

    _____

    _____

24. Place the following pharmacokinetic stages in order: metabolism, absorption, liberation, elimination, and distribution.

    _____

    _____

25. Describe drug *half-life*.

    _____

26. List three environmental poisons that are tested in toxicology.

    _____

    _____

    _____

Procedure 9-1: Assisting With Urine Collection for Drug Screening

Person evaluated _____   Date _____

Evaluated by _____   Score/Grade _____

Outcome goal	To assist with urine collection for drug screening
Conditions	Supplies required: - Urine drug screening collection kit with specimen cup with temperature indicator - Urine specimen containers to be sent to the laboratory - Plastic sealable pouch for the two urine specimen containers, chain-of-custody documents - Personal protective equipment
Standards	Required time: 15 minutes Performance time: _____ Total possible points = _____ Points earned = _____
Evaluation Rubric Codes: **S** = Satisfactory, meets standard **U** = Unsatisfactory, fails to meet standard	
NOTE: Steps marked with an asterisk (*) are critical to achieve required competency.	

Preparation	Scores	
	S	**U**
1. Explain to the patient the purpose of the test and the procedure to be followed for a midstream clean-catch specimen collection.		
- Had patient state name.		
- Obtained a signed consent form from the patient.		
- Compared with requisition.		

Procedure	Scores	
	S	**U**
2. Sanitized hands and put on gloves and face mask.		
3. A trained professional must witness the voiding of at least 50 mL of urine into the specimen cup provided in the urine collection drug kit.		
4. Originate the chain-of-custody document at the time of the sample collection. The person who witnessed the voiding must sign the document, as must every other person who handles the sample.		
5. After the collection, verify the temperature of the urine as seen on the indicator at the bottom of the cup, and document it. *Note:* If the temperature of the urine specimen is out of range (too cold), a second specimen must be collected. If the donor refuses to provide the second specimen under direct observation, the collection would be considered a "refusal to test."		
*6. Transfer the specimen to the two containers that must be labeled with the following information: - Full name of the patient - Date and time of collection - Your initials - Initials of the witnessing officer		
7. Place the two sample containers into the sealed plastic pouch, mark it with a notary-style seal or with tamper-proof tape to protect the integrity of the sample, and send the specimen to the toxicology laboratory.		
8. If you are trained and qualified to do the testing, proceed with the testing according to laboratory and state regulations.		

189

Follow-up	Scores	
	S	U
9. After the initial and confirmatory testing is complete, mark the urine sample, reseal it, and securely store it for a minimum of 30 days or for the length of time specified by laboratory protocols.		
10. Completed proper documentation on patient chart (see below).		
11. Proper disposal and disinfection.		
- Disinfected test area and instruments according to OSHA guidelines.		
- Disposed of regulated medical waste (e.g., gloves, tongue depressor) in biohazard bags.		
*12. Sanitized hands.		
Total Points per Column		

Patient Name: _____

Patient Chart Entry: (Include when, what, how, why, any additional information, and the signature of the person charting.)

_____

_____

_____

Procedure 9-2: Assisting With Blood Collection for Alcohol Testing

Person evaluated _____   Date _____

Evaluated by _____   Score/Grade _____

Outcome goal	To assist with blood collection for drug screening
Conditions	Supplies required: - Gray-topped Vacutainer tubes - Venipuncture needle and holder (or syringe and transfer device) - Nonvolatile disinfectant (e.g., benzalkonium [Zephiran], aqueous thimerosal [Merthiolate]) - Gauze - Tourniquet - Gloves - Legally authorized transportation envelope, container, or plastic pouch
Standards	Required time: 15 minutes Performance time: _____ Total possible points = _____ Points earned = _____

Evaluation Rubric Codes:
S = Satisfactory, meets standard   **U** = Unsatisfactory, fails to meet standard

NOTE: Steps marked with an asterisk (*) are critical to achieve required competency.

Patient Preparation	Scores	
	S	U
1. An officer of the law is present to act as a witness to the procedure.		
2. The patient probably is likely still to be under the influence of alcohol, so explain what you will be doing in as concise a manner as possible. *Note:* Do not allow yourself to become irritated by the speech or mannerisms of the patient. Treat the patient with the respect and dignity with which you treat all patients.		

Blood Collection Procedure	Scores	
	S	U
Note: The Department of Justice for each state has established uniform standards for the collection, handling, and preservation of blood samples used for alcohol testing. If you are authorized to obtain specimens for forensic analysis, check your laboratory's procedure manual so that you perform the collection *exactly* as required by the uniform standards established for your state.		
3. Sanitize hands, and apply gloves.		
4. Prepare the draw site using Zephiran, aqueous Merthiolate, or another aqueous disinfectant. *Do not use alcohol or other volatile organic disinfectants to clean the skin site.*		
5. Complete the blood draw, filling both tubes with sufficient blood to permit duplicate blood alcohol determinations.		
6. Label the two gray-stoppered tubes with the following information: - Full name of the patient - Date and time of collection - Your initials - Initials of the witnessing officer		

7. Give the labeled blood samples to the witnessing officer, who will immediately complete the required information on the transportation envelope, container, or plastic pouch. The officer will then seal it securely. Information on the envelope or container should include the following:
  - The full name of the patient
  - Whether the patient is alive or dead
  - The submitting agency
  - The geographic location where the blood was drawn (e.g., hospital, clinic, jail)
  - The name of the person drawing the blood sample
  - The date and time the blood sample was drawn
  - The signature of the witnessing officer		

8. After the envelope or container is sealed, it must not be opened except for analysis. Each person who is subsequently in possession of the sealed sample must sign his or her name in the space provided on the envelope or container (chain of custody). The integrity of the sample must be safeguarded.		
9. Remove gloves, and wash hands.		
Total Points per Column		

Patient Name: _____

Patient Chart Entry: (Include when, what, how, why, any additional information, and the signature of the person charting.)

_____

_____

_____

9.2 (continued): AFFECTIVE (BEHAVIORAL) COMPETENCY:
V.A1. DEMONSTRATE EMPATHY, ACTIVE LISTENING, AND NONVERBAL COMMUNICATION SKILLS; V.A3. DEMONSTRATE RESPECT FOR INDIVIDUAL DIVERSITY

Explanation: Student must achieve a **minimum score of 3 in each category** to achieve competency.

Demonstrating respect for individual diversity is extremely important when working with a diverse patient population. **Empathy**: respects the individuality of the patient and attempts to see the person's health problem through his or her **eyes.** It is the key to creating a caring, therapeutic environment. Three processes are involved in **active listening:** restatement, reflection, and clarification. Much of what we communicate to our patients is conveyed through the use of conscious or unconscious body language. Our **nonverbal actions**, such as gestures, facial expressions, and mannerisms, express our true feelings. 90% of communication is nonverbal. Although the verbal message is an important method of delivering information, the **way** we deliver those words is how the patient will interpret them.

Some questions you should consider when communicating with a patient from a diverse background include:
- Is language an issue with your patient?
- Does the patient's culture, ethnic background, or religious beliefs influence the way he or she perceives disease and/or the role of healthcare workers?
- What strategies or techniques might minimize communication problems?
- Are community resources available that could facilitate therapeutic communication?

Approaches for Language Barriers
- Address the patient by his or her last name (e.g., Mrs. Martinez, Mr. Nguyen).
- Be courteous and use a formal approach to communication.
- Use gestures, tone of voice, facial expressions, and eye contact to emphasize appropriate parts of the discussion.
- Integrate pictures, handouts, models, and other aids that visually depict the material.
- Monitor the patient's body language—especially facial expression—for understanding or confusion.
- Use simple, everyday words as much as possible.
- Give the patient written instructions, preferably in their native language, for all procedures and treatments.
- Involve family members or use an interpreter.

Using the following case study, role-play with your partner how you would apply respect for diversity in this situation that requires extensive communication techniques. Demonstrate empathy, active listening, and nonverbal communication skills while performing the role-play exercise. Mr. Luigi Mario, a 61-year-old Italian patient, was brought to your office by an officer after an auto accident. The officer needs an alcohol blood sample to see if Mr. Mario was under the influence of alcohol during the accident. Mr. Mario is very anxious and emotional about the accident and doesn't understand what he needs to have done. He has limited understanding of English and has difficulty with vision, but the officer who brought him to the office today can act as an interpreter. Demonstrate how you will perform the pre-analytical steps of preparing Mr. Mario for a blood draw.

Procedure 9-2 (continued) Therapeutic Communications – Respect for Diversity

STUDENT NAME: _____ EVALUATOR _____ Date_____

Scoring Criteria (1 Through 4)	Excellent Evidence of Learning 4	Adequate Evidence of Learning 3	Limited Evidence of Learning 2	Unacceptable Evidence of Learning 1	Score Attempt 1	Score Attempt 2	Score Attempt 3
Demonstrates respect for individual diversity when explaining the procedure	Student demonstrates the highest level of respect for diversity	Student demonstrates mastery level of respect for diversity but does not apply all the principles	Student is developing competency of respect for diversity	Student demonstrates the main concepts of respect for diversity but does not perform them adequately			
Demonstrates empathy, active listening, and nonverbal communication skills	Student attends to all the patient's nonverbal behaviors throughout the interview	Student demonstrates mastery level of attending to nonverbal behaviors but does not apply the principles comprehensively	Student is developing competency in attending to nonverbal behaviors	Student does not perform attending to nonverbal behaviors adequately			
Recognizes the importance of the patient's education needs	Correctly identifies patient's diverse communication needs	Recognizes some of the patient's diverse communication needs	Limited recognition of patient's diverse communication needs	Fails to identify patient's diverse communication needs			
Analyzes the situation and applies an appropriate solution	Considers all of the patient factors before reaching a solution	Identifies most of the patient factors	Limited recognition of patient factors	Fails to identify significant patient factors			
Evaluates the patient's understanding of the interaction	Accurately assesses the patient's understanding of the interaction	Briefly considers the patient's understanding of the interaction	Limited consideration of the patient's understanding of the interaction	Fails to evaluate the patient's understanding of the interaction			

Instructor/Evaluator Comments

Procedure 9-3: Urine Drug Panel Testing Procedure

Person evaluated _____   Date _____

Evaluated by _____   Score/Grade _____

Outcome goal	To perform FDA-approved, CLIA-waived drug panel test following the most current OSHA safety guidelines and applying the correct quality control
Conditions	Supplies required: - Gloves - Test card with multiple test strips (five tests are on each side of the card) - Metal pouch containing test card that has been stored at 2°C to 30°C (check expiration date)
Standards	Required time: 10 minutes Performance time: _____ Total possible points = _____ Points earned = _____
Evaluation Rubric Codes: **S** = Satisfactory, meets standard **U** = Unsatisfactory, fails to meet standard	
NOTE: Steps marked with an asterisk (*) are critical to achieve required competency.	

Preparation: Preanalytical Phase	Scores	
	S	U
A. Test information		
- Kit method:		
- Manufacturer:		
- Proper storage (e.g., temperature, light): store the card at 2°C to 30°C (check expiration date)		
- Lot # of kit:		
- Expiration date:		
- Package insert or test flow chart available: yes no		
B. Specimen information		
- Type of specimen: **Fresh urine specimen or specimen that has been stored at 2°C to 8°C for up to 48 hours and then brought to room temperature.**		
C. Sanitize the hands, and apply gloves.		

Procedure: Analytical Phase	Scores	
	S	U
D. Performed/observed qualitative quality control		
- External liquid controls: positive negative		
- Internal control: (appears as a red line on test stick)		
E. Performed patient test		
1. Sanitize the hands, and apply gloves.		
2. Remove the test device from its protective pouch, and label it with the patient's identification. *Note*: If the specimen has been stored in the refrigerator, bring it to room temperature before opening to prevent condensation.		
3. Remove the cap from the end of the test card.		

195

	Scores	
	S	U

4. With the arrows pointing toward the urine specimen, immerse the strips of the test card vertically into the urine specimen for at least 10 to 15 seconds. **Immerse the strips to at least the level of the wavy lines on the strips but not above the arrows on the test card.**		
5. Place the test card on a nonabsorbent surface, and wait for the colored lines to appear.		
6.		
- Positive test result: One distinct pink band appears in the control region (C), with no line in the test region (T).		
- Negative test result: Two pink bands appear, with one pink band in the control region (C) and one pink band in the patient test region (T).		
- Invalid: Pink bands are absent from the control region. Repeat the test with a new device. If the problem persists, call for technical assistance.		

*Accurate Results _____ **Instructor Confirmation** _____

Follow-up: Postanalytical Phase	Scores	
	S	U
*F. Proper documentation		
1. On control/patient log: _____ yes _____ no		
2. Documented on patient chart (see below).		
3. Identified critical values and took appropriate steps to notify physician.		
- Expected values for analytes: negative		
G. Proper disposal and disinfection		
1. Disposed of all sharps in biohazard sharps containers.		
2. Disposed of all other regulated medical waste in biohazard bags.		
3. Disinfected test area and instruments according to OSHA guidelines.		
4. Sanitized hands after removing gloves.		
Total Points per Column		

Patient Name: _____

Patient Chart Entry: (Include when, what, how, why, any additional information, and the signature of the person charting.)

_____

_____

_____

10 Electrocardiography

VOCABULARY REVIEW

Match each definition with the correct term.

Cardiology Terms

_____ 1. The relaxation phase in the heart when there is no electrical activity within the cardiac muscle

_____ 2. Pattern of P, Q, R, S, T, and U waves on an ECG recording

_____ 3. The 10 "sensors" placed on the limbs and chest that detect the electrical activity of the heart

_____ 4. Tracings other than from the heart or lungs that interfere with the interpretation of the ECG recordings

_____ 5. Fast heart rate

_____ 6. Structures that receive blood from the body on the right side and from the lungs on the left side

_____ 7. The contraction phase of the heart when the cardiac muscle is being stimulated by electrical impulses

_____ 8. Sends out an electrical impulse that starts the heartbeat

_____ 9. A sequence of two phases: a contraction phase and a relaxation phase

_____ 10. A muscular wall that divides the right and left sides of the heart

_____ 11. Heart rhythm is within normal limits

_____ 12. Blood flowing to the body and back to the heart

_____ 13. Slow heart rate

_____ 14. Breast bone

_____ 15. Between the ribs

_____ 16. Blood flowing to the lungs and back to the heart

_____ 17. Collar bone

_____ 18. Tracings other than from the heart that interfere with the interpretation of the ECG or spirometer recordings

_____ 19. The two lower chambers of the heart that send blood to the lungs and the body.

A. bradycardia
B. systole
C. atria
D. ECG cycle
E. systemic circulation
F. septum
G. artifacts
H. cardiac cycle
I. diastole
J. electrodes
K. sinus rhythm
L. tachycardia
M. sinoatrial (SA) node
N. ventricles
O. intercostal
P. pulmonary circulation
Q. sternum
R. artifacts
S. clavicle

Heart Anatomy and the ECG

20. Blood enters the right and left _____ of the heart, and is pumped out of the heart by the right and left _____.

21. The cardiac cycle consists of a contraction phase known as _____ and a relaxation phase known as _____.

22. Identify the five electrical conduction structures in the heart and the heart chambers that contract as a result of electrical stimulation (see Fig. 10.3 in the textbook).

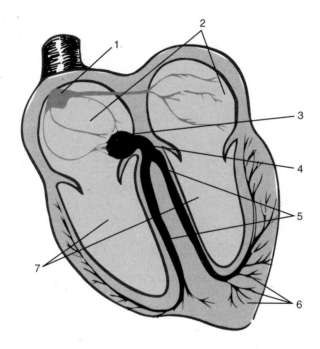

23. Who invented the first practical electrocardiogram? _____ What were his first three "leads" or tracings of the heart beating? _____. These leads required two limbs and were referred to as _____ leads.

24. How many electrodes are placed on the patient in the standard ECG? How many leads are recorded?

25. Label the nine components involved in recording an ECG tracing. (Note: Refer to Fig. 10.8 in the textbook.)

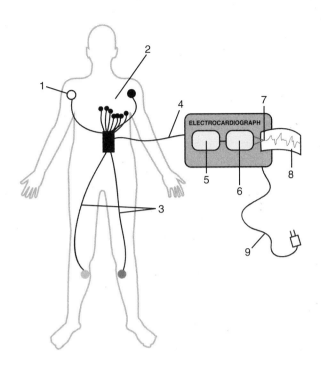

26. Match the following leads with their appropriate electrical descriptors:

_____ and _____ and ____ = V_1, V_2, V_3, V_4, V_5, and V_6 a. Augmented limb leads

_____ and _____ = I, II, and III   b. Unipolar leads (used twice)

_____ and _____ = aVR, aVF, and aVL   c. Standard limb leads

d. Chest leads

e. Bipolar leads

f. Precordial leads

27. Match the chest leads with their appropriate electrode placement

_____ V_1	a. Midway between the V_2 and V_4 positions
_____ V_2	b. 4th intercostal space on the left side of the sternum leads
_____ V_3	c. 5th intercostal space on the left midclavicular line
_____ V_4	d. Horizontal to V_4 at the left midaxillary line
_____ V_5	e. Horizontal to V_4 at the left anterior axillary line
_____ V_6	f. 4th intercostal space on the right side of the patient's sternum

Chapter **10 Electrocardiography**

28. Draw a standard pulse and one ECG tracing. Then label the waves: P, Q, R, S, and T. (Refer to Fig. 10.11 in the textbook.)

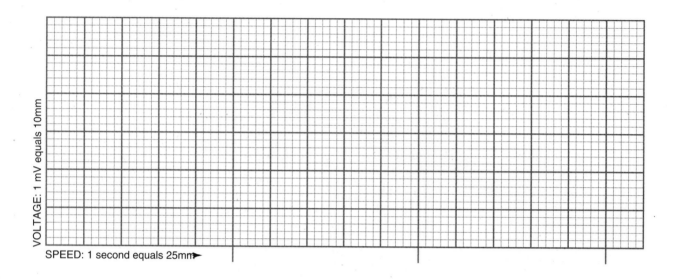

VOLTAGE: 1 mV equals 10mm

SPEED: 1 second equals 25mm

DIAGNOSTIC PROCEDURES

ECG Patient Preparations, Instructions, and Identification of Artifacts

29. Two ways to reduce a patient's anxiety about the ECG test include referring to it as a(n) _____ test and to the sticky electrodes as _____.

30. What should you do if a large patient does not have room on the examination table to rest his arms comfortably?

_____

31. Why should the patient remain still during the ECG recording?

_____

32. Write down the causes (or names) of the four artifacts seen on the ECG tracings below (A-D). Then match each artifact example with two ways to correct the artifact from the answers (a-h) below.

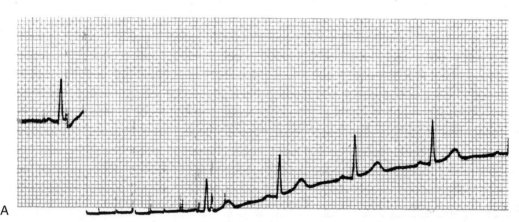

A

(Modified from Bonewit-West K: *Clinical procedures for medical assistants,* ed 9, St Louis, 2015, Saunders, with reference to Long BW: *Radiography essentials for limited practice,* ed 3, 2010, Saunders.)

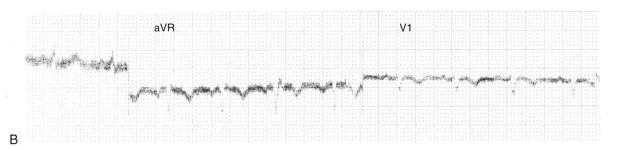

B

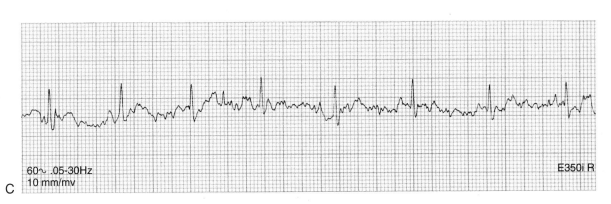

60~ .05-30Hz
10 mm/mv

E350i R

C

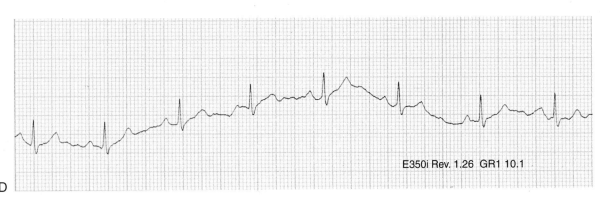

E350i Rev. 1.26 GR1 10.1

D

Name the four artifacts shown above on lines (A-D) below. Match the causes and ways to correct each of the listed artifacts using the lower case a. through h. answers below. (Note: Each listed artifact has two cause/corrections from the list of a-h below.)

A. _____ Causes/Corrections: _____ and _____

B. _____ Causes/Corrections: _____ and _____

C. _____ Causes/Corrections: _____ and _____

D. _____ Causes/Corrections: _____ and _____

a) Check if patient is comfortable and relaxed.
b) The electrode is not making contact because of hair on the legs or chest. Shave the site and reapply a new electrode.
c) Check if the patient cable or the lead wires are dangling and not supported.
d) Check if the power cord is running under the examination table.
e) The cable showing the interrupted pattern may be damaged and may need to be replaced.
f) Have the patient hold his or her breath for 15 seconds.
g) The patient has Parkinson's disease with involuntary muscle tremors in the limbs.
h) Check if high-voltage wiring is running parallel in the walls or overhead.

Chapter **10 Electrocardiography**

33. While recording the ECG, you see interference in leads II and III but not in lead I. What limb is causing the interference?

_____

_____

ADVANCED ELECTROCARDIOGRAPHY CONCEPTS

Ambulatory ECG Monitoring

34. List two portable ways a patient may monitor his or her ECG over time.

_____

_____

Cardiac Pathology and the ECG

35. Considering all the examples of atrial arrhythmias and ventricular arrhythmias, which is the most serious and life-threatening? Hint: Think of a heart attack that requires cardiopulmonary resuscitation (CPR) using a defibrillator.

_____

ELECTROCARDIOGRAPHY PROCEDURES:

See Procedure 10.1: Electrocardiography and Procedure 10.2: Holter Monitoring at the end of this workbook chapter.

Procedure 10.1: Electrocardiography

Person evaluated _____ Date _____

Evaluated by _____ Score/Grade _____

Outcome goal	To demonstrate the proper technique for preparing the patient and recording a diagnostic ECG
Conditions	Given the following supplies: - (Razor) - Alcohol - 10 disposable electrodes - Patient cable with lead wires - Power cord - Gown for the patient - ECG three-channel instrument or computerized ECG program to connect the patient cable
Standards	Required time: 20 minutes Performance time: _____ Total possible points = _____ Points earned = _____
Evaluation Rubric Codes: **S** = Satisfactory, meets standard **U** = Unsatisfactory, fails to meet standard	
NOTE: Steps marked with an asterisk (*) are critical to achieve required competency.	

Preparation: Preanalytical Phase	Scores S	Scores U
A. Test information		
- Burdick three-channel or Midmark computerized program		
- Lot # on disposable electrodes: _____		
- Expiration date on electrode package: _____		
- Instructions provided by ECG manufacturer: _____ yes _____ no		
B. Patient preparation		
1. Cleansed hands and prepared room with clean table paper, pillow, gown, and drape.		
2. Greeted the patient and confirmed identity while entering demographic data (i.e., patient's name, number, age, address). Instructed patient how to apply gown and provided privacy as they disrobed and put on gown.		
3. After returning, obtained the patient's vital signs and entered the vital signs into the computer.		
4. Prepared the 10 sites in the following routine order:		
- Prepare the lower limbs by dry shaving the inner calf muscles if necessary and then rubbing the areas with an alcohol swab to encourage circulation at the sites.		
- Prepare the upper outer limbs with the alcohol swab followed by locating the general areas for the chest leads and rubbing the areas with the alcohol swab.		
- Return to the legs and arms, and firmly press the electrode sensors with the tabs up on the legs and the tabs down on the arms. Check color-coded lead wires: green on RL, red on LL, black on LA, and white on RA.		

	Scores	

5. Relocated the actual chest sites by palpation and placed the electrodes in the following order:

- Locate the 4th intercostal space across to the right side of the patient's sternum then place the **V₁ electrode** with the tab down followed by the **V₂ electrode** directly across the sternum on the patient's left side (closest to you).

- Locate the V_4 lead location by following the 5th intercostal space and the intersecting midclavicular line and place the **V₄ electrode** on the site followed by the **V₃ electrode** midway between V_2 and V_4.

- Locate the last two lead locations by following a horizontal line around the ribs, based on the location of V_4, and place **V₅ electrode** on the intersecting anterior-lateral line of the chest and **V₆ electrode** at the intersecting midaxillary line of the chest.

- Methodically connect the numbered **V₁–V₆ lead wires** to each of their designated electrode locations.

Procedure: Analytical Phase	Scores	
	S	U
C. Performed/observed quality control by checking the speed of the paper was set at 25 mm/sec and the 0.1 mV caused a 10-mm rise on the recording.		
D. Performed the electrocardiography.		
1. Before starting the recording, the patient was informed that they needed to be very still and relaxed for about 15 seconds or so while the ECG is monitoring their heartbeats.		
2. Observed the three-channel ECG printout or the computer results for the following:		
- Check each lead in the tracing for unwanted artifacts and correct them if possible (i.e., AC interference, muscle tremors, wandering or interrupted baseline). Re-record another tracing if necessary.		
- Allow the physician to see the final product before disconnecting the patient from the ECG.		

*Accurate Results _____   Instructor Confirmation _____

Follow-up: Postanalytical Phase	Scores	
	S	U
*E. Proper documentation		
1. On control log _____ yes _____ no		
2. On patient log _____ yes _____ no		
3. Documented on patient chart (see below)		
F. Proper disposal and disinfection		
1. Removed and disposed of the electrodes and helped the patient to a sitting position.		
2. Instructed the patient to get dressed and that the physician would be sharing the findings with the patient.		
3. Disinfected test area and instruments according to OSHA guidelines.		
4. Sanitized hands.		
Totals Counts per Column		

Patient Name: _____

Patient Chart Entry: (Include when, what, how, why, any additional information, and the signature of the person charting.)

_____

_____

_____

Procedure 10.2: Holter Monitoring

Person evaluated _____ Date _____

Evaluated by _____ Score/Grade _____

Outcome goal	To demonstrate the proper technique to prepare a patient for Holter or ambulatory monitoring of ECG over time
Conditions	Given the following supplies: There are a variety of Holter monitoring systems in use. Most systems provide patient packets with all the supplies for preparing the patient included. The Midmark Holter packet consists of the following: - Five white electrodes to be placed on chest landmarks - Sterile razor for removing hair from sites - Abrasive pad to increase circulation at the sites - Alcohol swabs for removing oil and sweat - Patient cable with four lead wires and a green ground wire - New batteries for the monitor - Patient log for recording cardiac "events"
Standards	Required time: 20 minutes Performance time: _____ Total possible points = _____ Points earned = _____
Evaluation Rubric Codes: **S** = Satisfactory, meets standard **U** = Unsatisfactory, fails to meet standard	

Patient Preparation: Preanalytical Phase	Scores	
	S	U
1. Greeted the patient and confirmed identity while sanitizing hands.		
2. Explained procedure and how to disrobe (from the waist up with the gown opening in the front). Provided the patient with privacy.		
3. After returning, prepared the electrode sites by:		
a. Dry shaving hair (if necessary)		
b. Applying alcohol to remove lotions, oils, and dirt		
c. Rubbing the abrasive pad over the sites to increase circulation		
4. Noted the different configurations of where to place the **five** electrodes (and wires). Followed the manufacturer's diagram of the site locations or the physician's preference.		
5. Snapped the color-coded wires to their electrodes. One at a time, peeled the backing off of each sticky electrode with its colored lead wire and firmly pressed it on its appropriate prepared site. NOTE: Each Holter system provides its own diagram showing where each colored lead wire belongs.		
6. The wires coming from each electrode were looped and taped down with surgical tape or looped and held down by the lower sticky tab at the bottom of the electrode.		
7. Inserted the digital flashcard or tape into the Holter recorder. Placed the new batteries (provided in the supply kit) into the monitor, and connected the lead cable to the monitor.		

205

Procedure: Analytical Phase	Scores	
	S	U
8. Turned on the monitor and followed the manufacturer's directions for data input and quality control. Noted the start time on the monitor and wrote it in patient's log.		
9. Showed the patient the log book and how the monitor works and is stored in its pouch. Emphasized that the monitor and wires should not get wet.		
10. Instructed the patient to do the following in the log book (diary):		
- **Write down the activities** you do and exactly what time you do them using the clock on the Holter monitor screen. Activities include:		
- When you exert yourself		
- When you are at rest		
- When you eat		
- When you take medications		
- When you have bowel movements		
- **Write down any symptoms** you have while you are wearing the monitor, such as:		
- Chest pain		
- Shortness of breath		
- Lightheadedness		
- Skipped heartbeats		
- The physician will be comparing the data from the Holter monitor recorder with your diary, which will help diagnose your condition.		
11. Explained how long the patient will need to wear the monitor. (It may vary from 12 hours to 3 days or more based on the physician's order.)		
12. Documented in the patient record that all the above instructions were provided and when the patient was told to return.		

Follow-up: Postanalytical Phase	Scores	
	S	U
13. Performed the following when the monitoring period was over and the patient returned with the Holter monitor and the diary:		
- Checked to ensure entries were made in the log (diary).		
- Turned off and disconnected the monitor per manufacturer's instructions.		
- Disconnected the cable from the monitor.		
- Removed the monitor from the pouch.		
- Carefully removed electrodes from patient and the lead wires and discarded.		
- Cleaned the patient's chest of any residual gel from the electrodes.		
- Removed and discarded the batteries from the monitor.		
- Removed the flashcard/tape from the monitor and diary and turned it in for interpretation.		
- Cleaned Holter monitor and patient cable with lead wires for next patient.		

14. Documented on patient chart (see below).		
15. Disinfected test area and instruments according to OSHA guidelines.		
Totals Counts per Column		

Patient Name: _____

Patient Chart Entry: (Include when, what, how, why, any additional information, and the signature of the person charting.)

_____

_____

_____

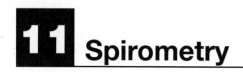
Spirometry

VOCABULARY REVIEW

Match each definition with the correct pulmonary term.

_____ 1. A test that measures how fast a person can exhale

_____ 2. Forced expiratory volume in the first second, expressed in liters

_____ 3. Forced vital capacity—the total volume of air exhaled in 6 seconds

_____ 4. Measurement of the volume and flow of air that is breathed

_____ 5. Chronic obstructive pulmonary disease

A. spirometry
B. peak flow rate
C. COPD
D. FEV$_1$
E. FVC

FUNDAMENTAL CONCEPTS

Anatomy of the Lungs and Spirometry

6. Match the following respiratory structures with their anatomical descriptions (A-D) and their associated obstructive disease descriptions (E-H). See Fig. 10.22.

Terminal bronchioles: _____ and _____	a. Primary, secondary, and tertiary bronchi
	b. Air sacs where gas exchanges take place
Lower respiratory tract: _____ and _____	c. Small airways capable of dilating or constricting
	d. Nasal cavity, pharynx, larynx, trachea
Upper respiratory tract: _____ and _____	e. Walls break down most commonly caused by smoking (emphysema)
	f. Infections such as colds, flu, allergies
Alveoli: _____ and _____	g. Muscles become swollen, and thick mucus forms, causing difficulty breathing in or out (asthma)
	h. Chronic condition typically caused by smoking, toxic fumes, or other irritants (bronchitis)

7. List the three steps of the spirometry "maneuver."

Step 1: _____

Step 2: _____

Step 3: _____

8. Write out the words represented for each abbreviated spirometry term represented on the "Volume/time chart" and the "Flow/Volume chart" seen on a spirometry report. (See Fig. 11.2 in textbook)

Volume/time chart (graph seen on the right side of the spirometry report):

A. FET _____

B. FVC _____

C. FEV_1_____

D. FEV_1/FVC ratio _____

Flow/volume chart—"peak flow chart" (seen in the graph on the left of the report):

E. PEF _____

F. $FEF_{25\%-75\%}$_____

9. Match each abbreviation above (A-F) with the description of the results they produce below (also see the spirometry report in Fig. 10.23 of the textbook). NOTE: The volume/time chart is on the right, and the flow/volume "peak flow chart" is on the left.

_____ breakdown of the peak flow chart on the left at 25%, 50%, and 75%

_____ vertical height of the line in the right chart, which shows how much air was exhaled in liters (NOTE: this will vary by patient based on age, size, gender, and race)

_____ highest point on the left graph representing maximum (peak) flow during the maneuver

_____ the forced volume expelled in the first second

_____ the horizontal length of the curved line, which shows how long the patient exhaled, in seconds (ideally the line should continue for 6 seconds)

_____ percentage ratio comparing the amount of air exhaled in the first second with the total volume expelled, predicted to be 80% to 90% in a healthy person

10. When calibrating the spirometer, how many liters are sent into the mouthpiece? _____ What are the two environmental factors that affect the spirometry reading?

_____ and _____

DIAGNOSTIC SPIROMETRY PROCEDURES

Spirometer Patient Preparations, Instructions, and Identification of Artifacts

11. List the three things a patient should do to prepare for a spirometry test.

_____

_____

_____

12. When coaching a patient during spirometry, indicate with a "P" if the feedback statement is positive and an "N" if the feedback statement is negative.

_____	"Keep your eyes on the screen."
_____	"You didn't blow long enough."
_____	"You're not putting the mouthpiece far enough into your mouth."
_____	"I need you to blow out really hard."
_____	"Don't look away."
_____	"You didn't blow hard enough."
_____	"I need you to blow until I say stop."
_____	"I need you to seal you lips firmly around the mouthpiece so all your breath is captured."

13. What can be done to help the patient keep blowing for the full 6 seconds of the maneuver?

_____

14. If the patient shows signs of airway obstruction, the physician may order a post-bronchodilator test. Why?

_____

ADVANCED SPIROMETRY CONCEPTS

Peak Expiratory Flow Screening and Monitoring

15. The maneuver for using the ambulatory peak flow monitor (PFM) has only two steps. Describe these steps.

Step 1:

_____

_____

Step 2:

_____

_____

16. When using a peak flow meter in the ambulatory setting, the patient's results are compared with those of other individuals with the same three demographics. List them.

1. _____

2. _____

3. _____

17. List the symptoms and physical findings seen in a child experiencing an asthmatic attack and respiratory distress.

_____

_____

_____

18. When an asthmatic child is measuring and recording his peak flow meter results daily, it is important to explain the significance of the three colored "zones." Briefly state what each zone represents.

Green zone: _____

Yellow zone: _____

Red zone: _____

19. List the three ways asthmatic patients may find relief when experiencing respiratory distress.

1. _____

2. _____

3. _____

20. List the two basic types of drug therapies used in asthma treatment. (Hint: One reduces swelling and mucus formation, and the other relaxes the muscles in the bronchioles.)

_____

_____

21. Describe the difference between a metered dose inhaler and a nebulizer for the delivery of medications.

_____

_____

_____

22. Why should you be familiar with administering nebulizer and oxygen treatments in the ambulatory setting?

_____

BEHAVIORAL 11-1: Instructing a Patient How to Perform the Spirometry Maneuver in Procedure 11-1, or Explaining and Demonstrating How to Perform the Peak Expiratory Flow Maneuver in Procedure 11-2

Work in groups of three students each. Each student will play a different role in the two instructional procedures (Spirometry, and/or Peak Expiratory Monitoring). When acting as the medical assistant giving the instructions, sign the top line below and have two other students sign in with their respective roles (patient or evaluator).

Medical assisting student being evaluated _____

Student playing the role of the patient _____

Student evaluator: _____(check off both the Behavioral and the Procedural sections based on your observations and then sign and date the forms)

COMPETENCY:	**I.A.3. Show awareness of a patient's concerns related to Procedure 11-2**: Instructing a Patient How to Perform the Spirometry Maneuver, **or Procedure 11-3**: Explaining and Demonstrating How to Perform the Peak Expiratory Flow Maneuver				
OBJECTIVE(s):	Given the conditions, and provided the necessary supplies, the student will demonstrate awareness of patient concerns as they provide patient care in a role-play scenario for a student-partner.				
TIME FRAME:	15 minutes				
GRADING:	**PASS = 100% accuracy.** All steps must be completed as written for "**PASS.**" Students are permitted two (2) graded attempts. **Grading Instructions:** When step is performed as written, record a "✓" for "**PASS.**" When step is omitted and/or there is an error in written procedure, record instructor initials for "**FAIL.**" Procedure must be repeated.				

		GRADED ATTEMPT 1		GRADED ATTEMPT 2	
STEP #	**PROCEDURE (check the procedure you performed as a medical assistant student)** ___ **1. Spirometry test instruction (11.2)** ___ **2. Peak Expiratory Flow Monitoring (11.3)**	**PASS**	**FAIL**	**PASS**	**FAIL**
Example	Instructions to evaluator: Student **completes step** as written, record "✓" Student **omits step or performs it in error,** record initials	✓	**ZH**		
1.	Gathered supplies and reviewed the new or established patient's medical history form.				
2.	Correctly prepared the patient: ■ Greeted the patient, introduced self, escorted him/her to exam room, and verified name. ■ Made appropriate eye contact with the patient ■ Established a professional and empathetic atmosphere ■ Explained procedure to patient				
3.	Responded to patient concerns: ■ Showed empathy toward patient ■ Assured patient concerns are understood by repeating them and verifying them with patient ■ Explained procedure again to ensure patient understanding ■ Answered any questions from patient ■ Assured patient that procedure is necessary ■ Provided necessary follow-up contact information				

Evaluator signature _____   MA student signature _____

Date _____

Procedure 11.1: Spirometry

Person evaluated _____ Date _____

Evaluated by _____ Score/Grade _____

Outcome goal	To demonstrate the proper technique for preparing the patient and recording a diagnostic spirometer test
Conditions	Given the following supplies: - Spirometer instrument or computer connected to printers - A disposable sterile mouthpiece connected to the plastic tubing on the spirometer (take care not to touch the area where the patient's mouth will be placed) - A nose clip (based on the physician's preference) - A chair for the patient to sit on if he or she becomes fatigued during the maneuver - Disposable gloves, to be worn during and after the patient's test to avoid the transmission of possible respiratory viruses and other respiratory pathogens - 3-liter syringe for calibrating the spirometer
Standards	Required time: 20 minutes Performance time: _____ Total possible points = _____ Points earned = _____

Evaluation Rubric Codes:
S = Satisfactory, meets standard   **U** = Unsatisfactory, fails to meet standard

NOTE: Steps marked with an asterisk (*) are critical to achieve required competency.

Preparation: Preanalytical Phase	Scores	
	S	U
A. Test information		
- Midmark computerized spirometer program (or other)		
- Lot # on disposable mouthpiece: _____		
- Instructions provided by ECG manufacturer: _____ yes _____ no		
B. Patient preparation		
1. Called the patient into the room and sanitized hands while confirming the patient's identity by asking for three identifiers: spell last name; give date of birth; and provide one more identifier, such as phone number, address, or driver's license.		
2. Entered the following data into the spirometer: patient's name, ID number, age, height, weight, gender, and race. NOTE: All this information is critical for the spirometer to produce the appropriate "predicted" results.		
3. Confirmed when the patient last took bronchodilator medication and if he or she smoked and noted it on the chart. Also, if appropriate, checked to make sure the patient does not have loose dentures that would interfere with the breathing maneuver.		
4. Explained and demonstrated the three steps of the maneuver using a mouthpiece that is not connected to the spirometer:		
- **Fully inflated** lungs and then held your breath while sealing lips around the mouthpiece.		
- **Fully exhaled** into the mouthpiece as fast and as hard as possible.		
- **Gave full effort** to exhale the remaining air in lungs for another 5 seconds without inhaling until the time is up.		
5. Showed and explained the importance of standing upright during the maneuver and that the patient will have a minute to rest and sit between a minimum of three attempts.		

Procedure: Analytical Phase	Scores	
	S	U
C. Performed/observed quality control by running a test using the 3-liter calibration syringe with results falling within +/− 3% of 3 liters.		
D. Performed the spirometer test.		
1. Coached the patient as he or she performed the maneuver. Watched patient, making sure he or she performed all three steps: inspiration, rapid exhalation, and extended exhalation. Praised what the patient did well and communicated positive ways to improve the next maneuver. Did not give negative feedback.		
2. Observed the two graph results and the spirometer feedback after each maneuver and had the patient rest for a minute:		
- The *time/volume curve* should have shown a sharp rise within the first second and then a slight steady rise for the next 2 to 6 seconds.		
- The *volume/flow curve* should have shown a fast rise in the beginning of the graph with a gradual curve downward that ends on the baseline.		
3. Repeated at least three maneuvers, until the patient was able to perform two reproducible results.		
*Accurate Results _____ Instructor Confirmation _____		

Follow-up: Postanalytical Phase	Scores	
	S	U
*E. Proper documentation		
1. On control log _____ yes _____ no		
2. On patient log _____ yes _____ no		
3. Documented on patient chart (see below)		
F. Proper disposal and disinfection		
1. Discarded the patient's mouthpiece and gloves in biohazard container and sanitized hands.		
2. Instructed the patient to get dressed and that the physician would be sharing the findings with the patient.		
3. Disinfected test area and instruments according to OSHA guidelines.		
Totals Counts per Column		

Patient Name: _____

Patient Chart Entry: (Include when, what, how, why, any additional information, and the signature of the person charting.)

_____

_____

_____

Procedure 11.2: Peak Expiratory Flow Monitoring

Person evaluated _____ Date _____

Evaluated by _____ Score/Grade _____

Outcome goal	To demonstrate the proper technique for measuring a patient's peak expiratory flow using a peak flow meter
Conditions	Given the following supplies: - Height/weight scale - New or sterilized peak flow meter - Additional peak flow meter for demonstrating maneuver - Daily monitoring chart
Standards	Required time: 20 minutes Performance time: _____ Total possible points = _____ Points earned = _____

Evaluation Rubric Codes:
S = Satisfactory, meets standard   **U** = Unsatisfactory, fails to meet standard

NOTE: Steps marked with an asterisk (*) are critical to achieve required competency.

Preparation: Preanalytical Phase	Scores	
	S	U
A. Patient preparation		
1. Called the patient into the room and sanitized your hands while confirming the patient's identity by asking for three identifiers: spell last name; give date of birth; and provide one more identifier, such as phone number, address, or driver's license.		
2. Confirmed when the patient last took bronchodilator medication and if he or she had a heavy meal in the last 4 hours.		
3. Measured patient's height in inches and confirmed patient's age (to compare with proper demographic group if it is a screening test).		
4. Explained and demonstrated the two steps of the maneuver using a demo peak flow meter:		
- **Fully inflated** lungs and then held your breath while sealing lips around the mouthpiece.		
- **Fully exhaled** into the mouthpiece as fast and as hard as possible.		
5. Showed and explained the importance of standing upright during the maneuver and that the patient will have a minute to rest and sit between a minimum of three attempts.		

Procedure: Analytical Phase	Scores	
	S	U
B. Taught the patient as follows:		
1. Before each use, make sure the sliding pointer on the peak flow meter is reset to the zero mark.		
2. Stand up straight, and remove chewing gum or any food from your mouth.		
3. Take a deep breath and put the mouthpiece in your mouth. Seal your lips and teeth tightly around the mouthpiece.		
4. Record the number where the sliding pointer has stopped on the scale.		
5. Reset the pointer to zero. Repeat this routine three times. You will know you have done the technique correctly when the three readings are close together.		

217

6. Record the highest of the three readings on a graph or in a notebook. This is called the *"best effort."*		
7. Use the peak flow meter once a day or as directed by your physician. Measure peak flows about the same time each day. A good time might be when you first wake up or at bedtime.		
C. Tested the patient as follows:		
8. Coached the patient as he or she performed the maneuver. Watched the patient to make sure both steps were performed: inspiration and rapid exhalation. Praised what the patient did well and communicated positive ways to improve the next maneuver. Did not give negative feedback.		
9. **If the patient is taking a screening test:** Located the patient's predicted value on the Peak Expiratory Flow Rate table (Table 11.1, found in your textbook). Divided the predicted value into the patient's result. If less than 80% of the predicted value, patient may need further evaluation.		
10. **If the patient is prescribed daily peak flow monitoring:** Determined the patient's "best effort" reading from three attempts. The personal best value is used as a baseline for routine measurements. Showed the patient the daily peak flow chart at the end of this procedure, where the patient will enter daily results. Explained the importance of noting the three colored zones: green = good, yellow = contact the physician, red = danger, seek proper care.		

Quality Control	S	U
D. Made the patient aware of the following issues that prevent accurate readings and how to correct them:		
- Coughing during the maneuver will require the maneuver to be repeated.		
- Poor seal around the mouthpiece while performing the procedure will give false low readings.		
- Taking asthma medication before the peak flow meter (especially bronchodilator medication) will open the airways and give a false high reading.		
- A dirty meter will not record accurately.		
- Blocking the mouthpiece with the tongue will give a false low reading.		
- Using a different type or brand of peak flow meter will cause the measurements to vary among brands and types of meters.		

*Accurate Results _____ **Instructor Confirmation** _____

Follow-up: Postanalytical Phase	Scores	
	S	U
*E. Proper documentation		
1. On control log _____ yes _____ no		
2. On patient log _____ yes _____ no		
3. Documented on patient chart (see below)		
F. Proper disposal and disinfection		
- Disinfected test area and instruments according to OSHA guidelines.		
Totals Counts per Column		

Patient Name: _____

Patient Chart Entry: (Include when, what, how, why, any additional information, and the signature of the person charting.)

_____

_____

_____

Appendix: Forms for Documenting Safety, Quality Assurance, CLIA Compliance, Sample Health Assessment Form, and Behavioral and Professional Evaluation Forms

CONTENTS

219

LABORATORY TECHNICIAN RESPONSIBILITIES IN CLASSROOM LABORATORY

Full Name of Tech	Official Initials	Temp Check Date	Disinfected Counters	Other

221

MONTHLY LABORATORY MAINTENANCE LOG

Medical Clinic

Daily Maintenance Control Chart

Month		Year							

Day	Daily					Monthly		By
	Refrig	Freezer	Room	Incubator	Bleach	Eye Wash	Shower	
	2-8°C	−0-20°C	15-30°C	34-36°C	Counters	Checked	Checked	
1								
2								
3								
4								
5								
6								
7								
8								
9								
10								
11								
12								
13								
14								
15								
16								
17								
18								
19								
20								
21								
22								
23								
24								
25								
26								
27								
28								
29								
30								
31								

Comments

Exposure Event Number_____

Blood and Body Fluid Exposure Report Form

Facility name: _____

Name of exposed worker: Last: _____ First: _____ ID#: _____

Date of exposure: _____ / _____ / _____   Time of exposure: _____ : _____ **AM   PM** (Circle)

Job title/occupation: _____   Department/work unit: _____

Location where exposure occurred: _____

Name of person completing form: _____

Section I. Type of Exposure *(Check all that apply.)*

- [ ] **Percutaneous (Needle or sharp object that was in contact with blood or body fluids)**
  (Complete Sections II, III, IV, and V.)

- [ ] **Mucocutaneous** *(Check below and complete Sections III, IV, and VI.)*
  ___ **Mucous Membrane**   ___ **Skin**

- [ ] **Bite** *(Complete Sections III, IV, and VI.)*

Section II. Needle/Sharp Device Information
(If exposure was percutaneous, provide the following information about the device involved.)

Name of device: _____   [ ] Unknown/Unable to determine

Brand/manufacturer: _____   [ ] Unknown/Unable to determine

Did the device have a sharps injury prevention feature, i.e., a "safety device"?

[ ] Yes   [ ] No   [ ] Unknown/Unable to determine

If yes, when did the injury occur?

[ ] Before activation of safety feature was appropriate   [ ] Safety feature failed after activation

[ ] During activation of the safety feature   [ ] Safety feature not activated

[ ] Safety feature improperly activated   [ ] Other: _____

Describe what happened with the safety feature, e.g., why it failed or why it was not activated: _____

_____

Section III. Employee Narrative *(Optional)*

Describe how the exposure occurred and how it might have been prevented:

_____

_____

_____

NOTE: This is not a CDC or OSHA form. This form was developed by CDC to help healthcare facilities with detailed exposure information that is specifically useful for the facilities' prevention planning. Information on this page (#1) may meet OSHA sharps injury documentation requirements and can be copied and filed for purposes of maintaining a separate sharps injury log. Procedures for maintaining employee confidentiality must be followed.

(Centers for Disease Control and Prevention,
http://www.cdc.gov/sharpssafety/pdf/AppendixA-7.doc)

223

Section IV. Exposure and Source Information

A.   **Exposure Details:** *(Check all that apply.)*

     1.   **Type of fluid or material (For body fluid exposures <u>only</u>, check which fluid in adjacent box.)**

         ☐ Blood/blood products

         ☐ Visibly bloody body fluid*

         ☐ Non-visibly bloody body fluid*

         ☐ Visibly bloody solution (e.g., water used to clean a blood spill)

> ***Identify which body fluid**
>
> | | | |
> |---|---|---|
> | ___ Cerebrospinal | ___ Urine | ___ Synovial |
> | ___ Amniotic | ___ Sputum | ___ Peritoneal |
> | ___ Pericardial | ___ Saliva | ___ Semen/Vaginal |
> | ___ Pleural | ___ Feces/stool | ___ Other/Unknown |

     2.   **Body site of exposure.** *(Check all that apply.)*

         ☐ Hand/finger   ☐ Eye   ☐ Mouth/nose   ☐ Face

         ☐ Arm   ☐ Leg   ☐ Other (Describe:_____)

     3.   **If percutaneous exposure:**

         Depth of injury *(Check only one.)*

         ☐ Superficial (e.g., scratch, no or little blood)

         ☐ Moderate (e.g., penetrated through skin, wound bled)

         ☐ Deep (e.g., intramuscular penetration)

         ☐ Unsure/Unknown

         Was blood visible on device before exposure?   ☐ Yes   ☐ No   ☐ Unsure/Unknown

     4.   **If mucous membrane or skin exposure:** *(Check only one.)*

         Approximate volume of material

         ☐ Small (e.g., few drops)

         ☐ Large (e.g., major blood splash)

         If skin exposure, was skin intact?   ☐ Yes   ☐ No   ☐ Unsure/Unknown

B.   **Source Information**

     1.   **Was the source individual identified?**   ☐ Yes   ☐ No   ☐ Unsure/Unknown

     2.   **Provide the serostatus of the source patient for the following pathogens.**

	Positive	Negative	Refused	Unknown
HIV Antibody	☐	☐	☐	☐
HCV Antibody	☐	☐	☐	☐
HbsAg	☐	☐	☐	☐

     3.   **If known, when was the serostatus of the source determined?**

         ☐ Known at the time of exposure

         ☐ Determined through testing at the time of or soon after the exposure

Section V. Percutaneous Injury Circumstances

A.   **What device or item caused the injury?**

Hollow-bore needle

☐ Hypodermic needle

   __ Attached to syringe __ Attached to IV tubing
   __ Unattached

☐ Prefilled cartridge syringe needle

☐ Winged steel needle (i.e., butterfly type devices)

   __ Attached to syringe, tube holder, or IV tubing
   __ Unattached

☐ IV stylet

☐ Phlebotomy needle

☐ Spinal or epidural needle

☐ Bone marrow needle

☐ Biopsy needle

☐ Huber needle

☐ Other type of hollow-bore needle (type: ____)

☐ Hollow-bore needle, type unknown

Suture needle

☐ Suture needle

Glass

☐ Capillary tube

☐ Pipette (glass)

☐ Slide

☐ Specimen/test/vacuum

☐ Other: _____

Other sharp objects

☐ Bone chip/chipped tooth

☐ Bone cutter

☐ Bovie electrocautery device

☐ Bur

☐ Explorer

☐ Extraction forceps

☐ Elevator

☐ Histology cutting blade

☐ Lancet

☐ Pin

☐ Razor

☐ Retractor

☐ Rod (orthopaedic applications)

☐ Root canal file

☐ Scaler/curette

☐ Scalpel blade

☐ Scissors

☐ Tenaculum

☐ Trocar

☐ Wire

☐ Other type of sharp object

☐ Sharp object, type unknown

Other device or item

☐ Other: _____

B.   **Purpose or procedure for which sharp item was used or intended.**
(Check one procedure type and complete information in corresponding box as applicable.)

☐ Establish intravenous or arterial access (Indicate type of line.) ⟶

☐ Access established intravenous or arterial line
(Indicate type of line and reason for line access.) ⟶

☐ Injection through skin or mucous membrane
(Indicate type of injection.)

☐ Obtain blood specimen (through skin)
(Indicate method of specimen collection.)

☐ Other specimen collection

☐ Suturing

☐ Cutting

☐ Other procedure

☐ Unknown

Type of Line

— Peripheral   — Arterial
— Central   — Other

Reason for Access

— Connect IV infusion/piggyback
— Flush with heparin/saline
— Obtain blood specimen
— Inject medication
— Other: _____

Type of Injection

__ IM injection   __ Epidural/spinal anesthesia
__ Skin test placement   __ Other injection
__ Other ID/SQ injection

Type of Blood Sampling

__ Venipuncture   __ Umbilical vessel
__ Arterial puncture   __ Finger/heelstick
__ Dialysis/AV fistula site   __ Other blood sampling

C. **When and how did the injury occur? (From the left hand side of page, select the point during or after use that most closely represents when the injury occurred. In the corresponding right-hand box, select *one* or *two* circumstances that reflect how the injury happened.)**

☐ During use of the item ──────────────►

Select one or two choices:

___ Patient moved and jarred device
___ While inserting needle/sharp
___ While manipulating needle/sharp
___ While withdrawing needle/sharp
___ Passing or receiving equipment
___ Suturing
___ Tying sutures
___ Manipulating suture needle in holder
___ Incising
___ Palpating/exploring
___ Collided with coworker or other during procedure
___ Collided with sharp during procedure
___ Sharp object dropped during procedure

☐ After use, before disposal of item ──────────────►

Select one or two choices:

___ Handling equipment on a tray or stand
___ Transferring specimen into specimen container
___ Processing specimens
___ Passing or transferring equipment
___ Recapping (missed or pierced cap)
___ Cap fell off after recapping
___ Disassembling device or equipment
___ Decontamination/processing of used equipment
___ During cleanup
___ In transit to disposal
___ Opening/breaking glass containers
___ Collided with coworker/other person
___ Collided with sharp after procedure
___ Sharp object dropped after procedure
___ Struck by detached IV line needle

☐ During or after disposal of item ──────────────►

Select one or two choices:

___ Placing sharp in container:
    _ Injured by sharp being disposed
    _ Injured by sharp already in container
___ While manipulating container
___ Over-filled sharps container
___ Punctured sharps container
___ Sharp protruding from open container
___ Sharp in unusual location:
    _ In trash
    _ In linen/laundry
    _ Left on table/tray
    _ Left in bed/mattress
    _ On floor
    _ In pocket/clothing
    _ Other unusual location
___ Collided with coworker or other person
___ Collided with sharp
___ Sharp object dropped
___ Struck by detached IV line needle

☐ Other (Describe): _____

_____

_____

_____

☐ Unknown

Section VI. Mucous Membrane Exposures Circumstances

A. **What barriers were used by worker at the time of the exposure?** *(Check all that apply.)*

☐ Gloves ☐ Goggles ☐ Eyeglasses ☐ Face Shield ☐ Mask ☐ Gown

B. **Activity/Event when exposure occurred** *(Check one.)*

☐ Patient spit/coughed/vomited
☐ Airway manipulation (e.g., suctioning airway, inducing sputum)
☐ Endoscopic procedure
☐ Dental procedure
☐ Tube placement/removal/manipulation (e.g., chest, endotracheal, NG, rectal, urine catheter)
☐ Phlebotomy
☐ IV or arterial line insertion/removal/manipulation
☐ Irrigation procedure
☐ Vaginal delivery
☐ Surgical procedure (e.g., all surgical procedures including C-section)
☐ Bleeding vessel
☐ Changing dressing/wound care
☐ Manipulating blood tube/bottle/specimen container
☐ Cleaning/transporting contaminated equipment
☐ Other: _____
☐ Unknown

Comments: _____

_____

_____

_____

_____

_____

_____

_____

_____

GENERIC QUALITATIVE CONTROL AND PATIENT LOG (TEMPLATE)

Test: _____

Kit Name and Manufacturer: _____

Lot #: _____   **Expiration Date:** _____

Storage Requirements: _____   **Test Flow Chart:** _____

Date	Tech Initials	Specimen ID (Control/Patient)	Result (+ or −)	Internal Control Passed (Y or N)	Charted in Patient Record

Appendix: Forms for Documenting Safety, Quality Assurance

GENERIC QUANTITATIVE TEST CONTROL LOG (TEMPLATE)

Control Lot #: _____   Expiration Date: _____

Control Range: _____   Control Level: _____

Date	Tech	Result	Accept	Reject	Corrective Action

230

MONTHLY LEVEY-JENNING QC CHART

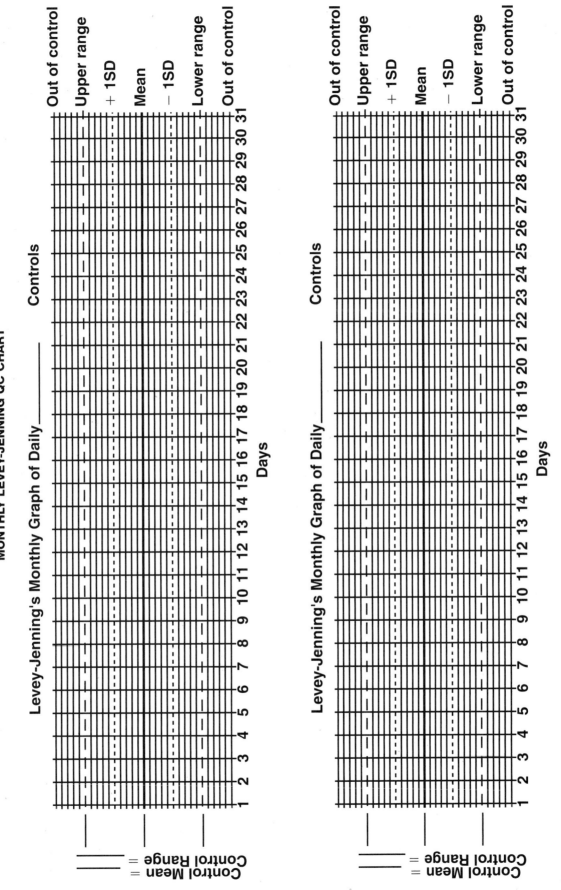

Appendix: Forms for Documenting Safety, Quality Assurance

URINE DIPSTICK QUALITY CONTROL LOG

DATE_____ URINE DIPSTICK CONTROL LEVEL _____ LOT #_____ EXPIRATION DATE_____

DATE	Reagent Strip — Lot # — Patient	DIPSTICK TESTS											CONFIRMATORY TESTS									ADD. TESTS		INITIAL
		Leukocytes	Nitrites	Urobilinogen	Protein	pH	Blood	Specific Gravity	Ketones	Bilirubin	Glucose	Protein	Method/Lot #	Ketones	Method/Lot #	Glucose	Method/Lot #	Bilirubin	Method/Lot #	hCG	Method/Lot #	Specific Gravity Refractometer	

233

URINE DIPSTICK PATIENT LOG

DATE	Reagent Strip		DIPSTICK TESTS												CONFIRMATORY TESTS								ADD. TESTS		INITIAL
	Lot#	Patient	Leukocytes	Nitrites	Urobilinogen	Protein	pH	Blood	Specific Gravity	Ketones	Bilirubin	Glucose	Protein	Method/Lot #	Ketones	Method/Lot #	Glucose	Method/Lot #	Bilirubin	Method/Lot #	hCG	Method/Lot #	Specific Gravity Refractometer	

Sample Device Preselection Worksheet

Type of Device: _____   Name: _____   Manufacturer: _____

Clinical Considerations	Does this consideration apply to this device?		If Yes, what is the level of importance?		
	No	Yes	High	Med	Low
Device use will require a change in technique (compared to conventional product).					
Device permits needle changes.					
Device permits reuse of the needle on the same patient during a procedure. (e.g., local anesthesia)					
Device allows easy visualization of flashback.					
Device allows easy visualization of medication.					
Other:					
Comment:					

Procedural Implications for Healthcare Provider

235

Clinical Considerations		Does this consideration apply to this device?		If Yes, what is the level of importance?		
		No	Yes	High	Med	Low
Patient Considerations	Device is latex free.					
	Device has potential for causing infection.					
	Device has potential for causing increased pain or discomfort to patients.					
	Other:					
	Comment:					
Scope of Device Use Considerations	Device can be used with adult and pediatric populations.					
	Specialty areas (e.g., OR, anesthesiology, radiology) can use the device.					
	Device can be used for all same purposes for which the conventional device is used.					
	Device is available in all currently used sizes.					
	Other:					
	Comment:					

Safety Considerations		Does this consideration apply to this device?		If Yes, what is the level of importance?		
		No	Yes	High	Med	Low
Method Activation	The safety feature does not require activation by the user.					
	The worker's hands can remain behind the sharp during activation of the safety.					
	Activation of the safety feature can be performed with one hand.					
	Other:					
	Comment:					
Characteristics of the Safety Feature	The safety feature is in effect during use in the patient.					
	The safety feature permanently isolates the sharp.					
	The safety feature is integrated into the device (i.e., does not need to be added before use).					
	A visible or audible cue provides evidence of safety feature activation.					
	The safety feature is easy to recognize and intuitive to use.					
	Other:					
	Comment:					

237

Other Considerations

Category	Other Considerations	Does this consideration apply to this device?		If Yes, what is the level of importance?		
		No	Yes	High	Med	Low
Availability	The device is available in all sizes currently used in the organization.					
	The manufacturer can provide the device in needed quantities.					
Service Provided	The company representative will assist with training.					
	Product materials are available to assist with training.					
	The company will provide free samples for evaluation.					
	The company has a history of being responsive when problems arise.					
	Comment:					
Practical Considerations	The device will **not** increase the volume of sharps waste.					
	The device will **not** require changes in the size or shape of sharps containers.					
	Other:					
	Comment:					

Centers for Disease Control and Prevention, "Sample Device Pre-Selection Worksheet," Sharps Injury Prevention Workbook, A-12, http://www.cdc.gov/sharpssafety/index.html.

SAMPLE DEVICE EVALUATION FORM

Product: _____   Date: _____

Department/unit: _____   Position/title: _____

1. **Number of times you used the device.**

   ☐ 1–5   ☐ 6–10   ☐ 11–25   ☐ 26–50   ☐ More than 50

2. **Please mark the box that best describes your experiences with the device. If a question is not applicable to this device, do not fill in an answer for that question.**

Factors	Strongly Disagree	Disagree	Neither Agree nor Disagree	Agree	Strongly Agree
Patient/Procedure Considerations					
a. Needle penetration **is** comparable to the standard device.	1	2	3	4	5
b. Patients/residents **do not** perceive more pain or discomfort with this device.	1	2	3	4	5
c. Use of the device **does not** increase the number of repeat sticks of patient.	1	2	3	4	5
d. The device **does not** increase the time it takes to perform the procedure.	1	2	3	4	5
e. Use of the device **does not** require a change in procedural technique.	1	2	3	4	5
f. The device is compatible with other equipment that must be used with it.	1	2	3	4	5
g. The device can be used for the same purposes as the standard device.	1	2	3	4	5
h. Use of the device **is not** affected by my hand size.	1	2	3	4	5
i. Age or size of patient/resident **does not** affect use of this device.	1	2	3	4	5
Experience with the Safety Feature					
j. Safety feature **does not** interfere with procedural technique.	1	2	3	4	5
k. The safety feature is easy to activate.	1	2	3	4	5
l. Safety feature **does not** activate before the procedure is completed.	1	2	3	4	5
m. Once activated, the safety feature remains engaged.	1	2	3	4	5
n. I **did not** experience any injury or *near miss* of injury with the device.	1	2	3	4	5

239

Appendix: Forms for Documenting Safety, Quality Assurance

Special Questions about This Device					
[To be added by health care facility]	1	2	3	4	5
	1	2	3	4	5
	1	2	3	4	5
Overall Rating					
Overall, the device is effective for patient and resident care and safety.	1	2	3	4	5

3. **Did you participate in training on how to use this product?**

   ☐ No *(Go to question 6.)*　　　　☐ Yes *(Go to next question.)*

4. **Who provided this instruction?** *(Check all that apply.)*

   ☐ Product representative　　　☐ Staff development personnel　　　☐ Other_____

5. **Was the training you received adequate?**

   ☐ No　　　　☐ Yes

6. **Was special training needed to use the product effectively?**

   ☐ No　　　　☐ Yes

7. **Compared with others of your gender, how would you describe your hand size?**

   ☐ Small　　　☐ Medium　　　☐ Large

8. **What is your gender?**

   ☐ Female　　　☐ Male

9. **Which of the following do you consider yourself to be?**

   ☐ Left-handed　　☐ Right-handed

10. **Please add any additional comments below.**

   _____

   _____

THANK YOU FOR COMPLETING THIS SURVEY

Please return this form to _____

(Centers for Disease Control and Prevention, Sample Device Evaluation Form, Sharps Injury Prevention Workbook, A-13; http://www.cdc.gov/sharpssafety/index.html)

LABORATORY REQUISITION
Biomedical Laboratories, Inc.
100 Main Street
Athens, Georgia 45760

☐ Fax	Send additional copy of report to:	( )
☐ Call	Client Number/Physician's Name	Phone/Fax number
☐ Mail	Physician's Address	City, State, Zip

Patient's Name (Last)	(First)	(MI)	Sex	Date of Birth MO DAY YEAR	Collection Time : AM PM	Fasting YES NO	Collection Date MO DAY YEAR

NPI/UPIN	Physician's ID #	Patient's SS #	Patient's ID #	Urine hrs/vol hrs___ vol___

PATIENT / RESP. PARTY

Physician's Name (Last, First)	Physician's Signature	Patient's Address	Phone
Medicare # (Include prefix/suffix)	☐ Primary ☐ Secondary	City	State ZIP
Medicaid #	State	Physician's Provider #	Name of Responsible Party (if different from patient)
Diagnosis/Signs/Symptoms in ICD-9 Format (Highest Specificity) REQUIRED		Address of Responsible Party (if different from patient)	APT #
		City	State ZIP

INSURANCE

Patient's Relationship to Responsible Party: ☐ 1–Self ☐ 2–Spouse ☐ 3–Child ☐ 4–Other

Performance Lab ☐ | Carrier | Group # | Employee # | Mem

Insurance Company Name	Plan	Carrier Code
Subscriber/Member #	Location	Group #
Insurance Address	Physician's Provider #	
City	State	ZIP
Employer's Name or Number	Insured SS # (If not patient)	Worker's Comp ☐ Yes ☐ No

I hereby authorize the release of medical information related to the service subscribed herein and authorize payment directed to LabCorp.

X _____ Patient's Signature _____ Date

MEDICARE ADVANCE BENEFICIARY NOTICE

I have read the ABN on the reverse. If Medicare denies payment, I agree to pay for the identified test(s).

X _____ Patient's Signature _____ Date

NOTE: WHEN ORDERING TESTS FOR WHICH MEDICARE OR MEDICAID REIMBURSEMENT WILL BE SOUGHT, PHYSICIANS SHOULD ONLY ORDER TESTS THAT ARE MEDICALLY NECESSARY FOR THE DIAGNOSIS OR TREATMENT OF THE PATIENT. COMPONENTS OF THE ORGAN OR DISEASE PANELS/COMBINATIONS PRINTED BELOW ARE SHOWN ON THE REVERSE SIDE AND MAY ALSO BE ORDERED INDIVIDUALLY BELOW. COMPONENTS MAY BE BILLED SEPARATELY PER CARRIER POLICY.

PROFILES (See reverse for components)

80049	Basic Metabolic Profile	SST
80054	Comp Metabolic Profile	SST
80051	Electrolyte Profile	SST
80058	Hepatic Profile	SST
80059	Hepatitis Profile	SST
80061	Lipid Profile	SST
80091	Thyroid Profile	SST
80055	Prenatal Profile	RED LAV
80072	Rheumatoid Profile	SST

HEMATOLOGY/COAGULATION

85025	CBC w Diff	LAV
85027	CBC w/o Diff	LAV
85014	Hematocrit	LAV
85018	Hemoglobin	LAV
85595	Platelet Count	LAV
85041	RBC Count	LAV
85048	WBC Count	LAV
85007	WBC Differential	LAV
89190	Nasal Smear, Eosin	Nasal Smear
85060	Pathologist Consult–Peripheral Smear	LAV
85651	Sed Rate	LAV
85610	Prothrombin Time (PT)	BLU
86900 86901	PT and PTT Activated	BLU
85730	PTT Activated	BLU

CHEMISTRY

82040	Albumin	SST
84075	Alkaline Phosphatase	SST
84460	ALT (SGPT)	SST
82150	Amylase, Serum	SST
84450	AST (SGOT)	SST

ALPHABETICAL TESTS CON'T

82607 82746	B₁₂ and Folate	SST
82250	Bilirubin, Total	SST
84520	BUN	SST
82310	Calcium	SST
82378	CEA	SST
82465	Cholesterol, Total	SST
82565	Creatinine	SST
82670	Estradiol	SST
82728	Ferritin, Serum	SST
82985	Fructosamine	SST
83001	FSH	SST
83001 83002	FSH and LH	SST
82977	GGT	SST
82947	Glucose, Plasma	GRY
82947	Glucose, Serum	SST
82950	Glucose, 2-hr. PP	SST
83036	Glycohemoglobin, Total	LAV
84703	hCG, Beta Subunit, Qual	SST
84702	hCG, Beta Subunit, Quant	SST
83718	HDL Cholesterol	SST
83036	Hemoglobin A₁c	LAV

SEROLOGY/IMMUNOLOGY

85610 85730	ABO and Rh	LAV
86038	Antinuclear Antibodies	SST
86677	Helicobacter pylori, IgG	SST
86706	Hep B Surface Antibody	SST
87340	Hep B Surface Antigen	SST
86803	Hep C Antibody	SST
86701	HIV Antibodies Serology	SST

ALPHABETICAL TESTS CON'T

83540	Iron, Total	SST
83540 83550	Iron and IBC	SST
83615	LDH	SST
83002	LH	SST
83690	Lipase	SER
83735	Magnesium, Serum	SST
84132	Potassium	SST
84146	Prolactin, Serum	SST
84153	Prostate-Specific Antigen	SST
84066	Prostatic Acid Phos	SST
84155	Protein, Total	SST
86431	Rheumatoid Arthritis Factor	SST
86592	RPR	SST
86762	Rubella Antibodies, IgG	SST
84295	Sodium	SST
84403	Testosterone	SST
84436	Thyroxine (T₄)	SST
84478	Triglycerides	SST
84480	Triiodothyronine (T₃)	SST
84443	TSH, High Sensitivity	SST
84550	Uric Acid	SST

TOXICOLOGY

80156	Carbamazepine (Tegretol®)	SER
80162	Digoxin	SER
80178	Lithium (Eskalith®)	SER
80184	Phenobarbital (Luminal®)	SER
80185	Phenytoin (Dilantin®)	SER
80198	Theophylline Toxicology	SER
80164	Valproic Acid (Depakene®)	SER

URINALYSIS

81003	Urinalysis	Microscopic on Positives	URN
81001	Urinalysis	with Microscopic	URN

MICROBIOLOGY   See Reverse Side
■ENDOCERVICAL ■ THROAT ■URINE ■STOOL ■ URETHRAL INDICATE SOURCE

87070	Aerobic Bacterial Culture	Bact Trnspt
87490 87590	Chlamydia/GC DNA Probe w/ Confirmation on Positives	Probe Trnspt
87490 87590	Chlamydia/GC DNA Probe Without Confirmation	Probe Trnspt
87490	Chlamydia DNA Probe	Probe Trnspt
87081	Genital, Beta-Hemolytic Strep Cult, Group B	Bact Trnspt
87070	Genital Culture, Routine	Bact Trnspt
87070	Lower Respiratory Culture	Steril Trnspt
87590	N. gonorrhoeae DNA Probe	Probe Trnspt
87015 87211	Ova and Parasites	O & P Kit
87081 X2 87045	Stool Culture	Fecal Trnspt
87081	Throat, Beta-Hemolytic Strep Cult, Group A	Bact Trnspt
87060	Upper Respiratory Culture, Routine	Bact Trnspt
87086	Urine Culture, Routine	Urn Cul Trnspt

Clinical Information/Comments

OTHER TESTS/INDIVIDUAL COMPONENTS

TEST #	TEST NAMES

LAB USE ONLY	STAT ☐998074	VENIPUNCTURE ☐998085	TRAVEL ☐998096	NON LABCORP ☐998239	VERBAL ORDER ☐998250	CHART ORDER ☐998261	HANDWRITTEN ☐998272	24 HR TUV ☐998283	PST/PSC #

CONTAINERS RECEIVED	SST SPUN	USST UNSPUN	SER SERUM	FRZ FRZ TRNSPT	RED RED	LAV LAVENDER	SLD SLIDE	BLU LT. BLUE	GRY GREY	GRN GREEN	RYB RYL BLU	YEL ACD	PLS PLASMA	URN URINE	24U 24 HR URINE	TA-U TART. ACID	FL FLUID	OT OTHER	BACT TRNSP	O & P KIT	PROBE TRNSP	URN CULT TRNSP	STERIL TRNSP	FECAL TRNSP	VIRAL TRNSP

300-0384

241

Appendix: Forms for Documenting Safety, Quality Assurance

SPECIMEN LOG SHEET

Date Sent	Tech Initials	PT. #	Doctor	Tests Ordered	Tubes Sent	Lab to Pick Up	Results Received

Quality Control Flow Chart for HemoCue

Regardless of the purpose, most clinical testing procedures have the same quality control requirements. If an instrument is used, there is usually a method to check its mechanical function. Often this is nothing more than an "optic check" or calibration strip supplied with the instrument to allow the user to determine whether the instrument is functional.

After determining that the instrument does indeed function, one then needs to prove that the reagents will perform as expected. Commonly, one uses a high and low value control sample. Look at the results. Are they within their expected ranges? If so, you can begin to test patients. If not, then it is time to do some troubleshooting.

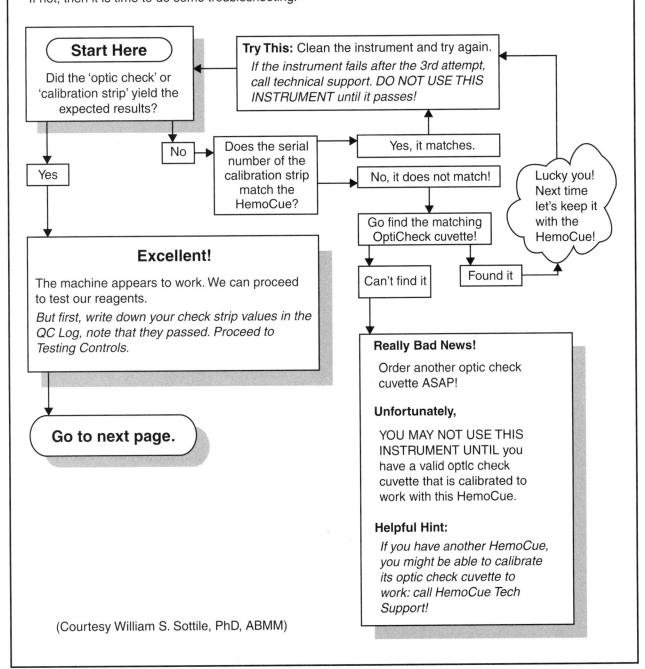

(Courtesy William S. Sottile, PhD, ABMM)

Appendix: Forms for Documenting Safety, Quality Assurance

HEMOGLOBIN QUALITY CONTROL LOG

Test: _____   Control Lot #: _____

Control Range: _____   For Low/Normal/High Control

Date	Tech	Result	Accept	Reject	Corrective Action

HEMOGLOBIN PATIENT LOG

Test: _____   Kit Lot #: _____

Expected Hemoglobin Values:

Adult males = 13.0–18 g/dL   Adult females = 11.0–16.0 g/dL

Infants = 10.0–14.0 g/dL   Children = Increase to adult

Date	Tech	Patient ID	Result	Charted

HEMATOCRIT QUALITY CONTROL LOG

Test: _____   Control Lot #: _____

Control Range: _____   For Low/Normal/High Control

Date	Tech	Slot #	Result	Accept	Reject	Corrective Action

Appendix: Forms for Documenting Safety, Quality Assurance

HEMATOCRIT PATIENT LOG

Expected Hematocrit Values:

Adult males = 42%–52%   Adult females = 36%–48%

Infants = 32%–38%   Children = Increase to adult

Date	Tech	Patient ID	Slot #	Result	Charted

ERYTHROCYTE SEDIMENTATION RATE PATIENT LOG

Expected ESR Values:

Adult males < 50 yr = 0–15 mm/hr   Adult females < 50 yr = 0–20 mm/hr

Adult males > 50 yr = 0–20 mm/hr   Adult females > 50 yr = 0–30 mm/hr

Date	Tech	Patient ID	Slot #	Time	Result	Charted

Appendix: Forms for Documenting Safety, Quality Assurance

COAGUCHEK PATIENT LOG

Coaguchek expected values for normal and therapeutic whole blood:

	INR	PT (seconds; see ranges in insert)
Normal	0.8–1.2	_____
Low anticoagulation	1.5–2.0	_____
Moderate anticoagulation	2.0–3.0	_____
High anticoagulation	2.5–4.0	_____

Date	Tech	Patient ID	INR	PT (seconds)	Charted

Appendix: Forms for Documenting Safety, Quality Assurance

GENERIC QUANTITATIVE TEST PROCEDURE (TEMPLATE)

Quantitative Test _____

Person evaluated _____   **Date** _____

Evaluated by _____   **Score/Grade** _____

Outcome goal:	
Conditions:	
Standards:	Required time = _____ minutes Performance time = _____
	Total possible points = _____ Points earned = _____

Evaluation Rubric Codes:
S = Satisfactory—Meets standard   **U** = Unsatisfactory—Fails to meet standard

NOTE: Steps marked with an asterisk (*) are critical to achieve required competency.

Preparation: Preanalytical Phase	Scores S	U
A. Test information		
- Kit or instrumental method: _____		
- Manufacturer: _____		
- Proper storage (e.g., temperature, light): _____		
- Lot number of kit or supplies: _____		
- Expiration date: _____		
- Package insert and/or test flow chart available: yes _____ no _____		
B. Specimen information		
- Type of specimen and its preparation (e.g., fasting, first morning):		
- Specimen container or testing device: _____		
- Amount of specimen: _____		
C. Personal protective equipment (PPE): _____		
D. Assembled all the above, sanitized hands, and applied PPE.		

Procedure: Analytical Phase	Scores S	U
E. Performed/observed quality control for A or B below.		
Quantitative testing controls		
- Calibration check: _____		
- Control levels: Normal _____ High _____ Low _____		

F. Performed patient test: Followed proper steps (see flow chart and list steps).	S	U
1.		
2.		
3.		
4.		
5.		
6.		
7.		
8.		
9.		
10.		
*Accurate Results _____ Instructor Confirmation _____		

Follow-up: Postanalytical	Scores	
	S	U
*G. Proper documentation		
1. On control log _____ yes _____ no		
2. On patient log _____ yes _____ no		
3. Documentation on patient chart (see below)		
4. Identified "critical values" and took appropriate steps to notify physician. EXPECTED VALUES FOR ANALYTE:		
H. Proper disposal and disinfection		
1. Disposed of all sharps into biohazard sharps containers.		
2. Disposed of all other regulated medical waste into biohazard bags.		
3. Disinfected test area and instruments according to OSHA guidelines.		
4. Sanitized hands after removing gloves.		
Column Totals		

Patient Name: _____

Patient Chart Entry: (Include when, what, how, why, any additional information, and the signature of the person charting.)

_____

_____

_____

GLUCOSE TEST CONTROL LOG

Control Lot #: _____   **Expiration Date:** _____

Control Range: _____   **Level: Low/Normal/High**

Date	Tech	Result	Accept	Reject	Corrective Action

GLUCOSE PATIENT LOG

Date	Tech	Patient	Result	Charted

HEMOGLOBIN A₁c PATIENT/CONTROL LOG

Date	Tech	Patient	Result	Charted

Appendix: Forms for Documenting Safety, Quality Assurance

CHOLESTECH LDX PATIENT/CONTROL LOG

Cassette Lot #: _____   Expiration Date: _____   LDX Serial #: _____

Date	Operator	Patient ID	Charted	TRG	TC	GLU	HDL	LDL	TC/HDL	ALT

HEMOCCULT PATIENT LOG

Date	Tech	Patient	Result

Appendix: Forms for Documenting Safety, Quality Assurance

I-STAT PATIENT/CONTROL LOG

Cartridge Lot #: _____   Expiration Date: _____   Serial #: _____

Date	Operator	Patient ID	Charted	Na	K	Cl	TCO$_2$	iCa	Glu	BUN	Crea	Hct	Hb	AnGap

Appendix: Forms for Documenting Safety, Quality Assurance

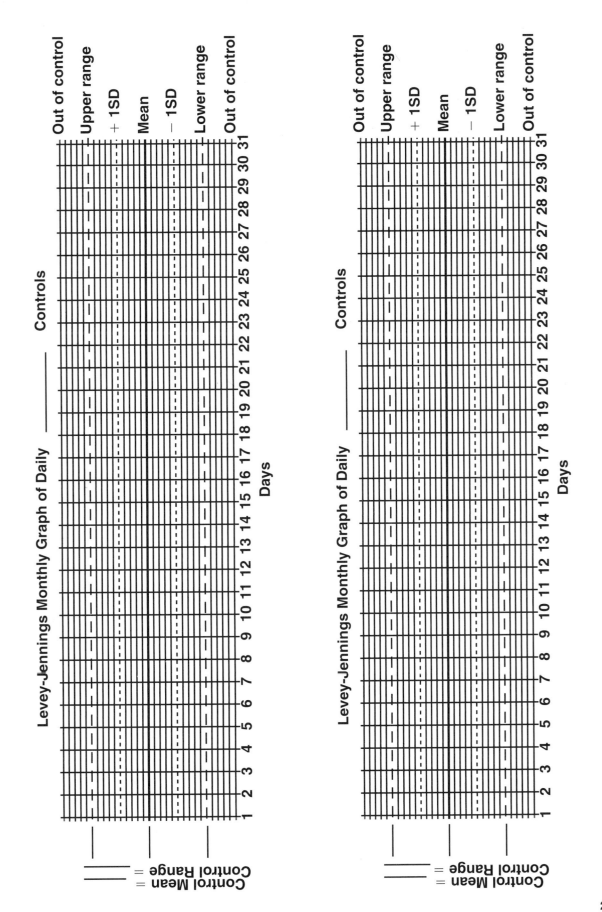

Appendix: Forms for Documenting Safety, Quality Assurance

QUALITATIVE CONTROL AND PATIENT LOG FOR IMMUNOLOGY AND MICROBIOLOGY TEST KITS (TEMPLATE)

Test: _____

Kit Name and Manufacturer: _____

Lot # _____   Expiration Date: _____

Storage Requirements: _____   Test Flow Chart: _____

Date	Tech Initials	Specimen ID (Control/Patient)	Result (+ or −)	Internal Control Passed (Y or N)	Charted in Patient Record

GENERIC QUALITATIVE TEST PROCEDURE (TEMPLATE)

Qualitative Test _____

Person evaluated _____ **Date** _____

Evaluated by _____ **Score/Grade** _____

Outcome goal:	
Conditions:	Supplies required:
Standards:	Required time = _____ minutes Performance time = _____
	Total possible points = _____ Points earned = _____

Evaluation Rubric Codes:
S = Satisfactory—Meets standard   **U** = Unsatisfactory—Fails to meet standard

NOTE: Steps marked with an asterisk (*) are critical to achieve required competency.

Preparation: Preanalytical Phase	Scores	
	S	**U**
A. Test information		
- Kit method:		
- Manufacturer:		
- Proper storage (e.g., temperature, light):		
- Lot number of kit: _____		
- Expiration date: _____		
- Package insert and/or test flow chart available: _____ yes _____ no		
B. Personal protective equipment		
C. Specimen information		

Procedure: Analytical Phase	Scores	
	S	**U**
D. Performed/observed qualitative quality control		
- External liquid controls: Positive _____ Negative _____		
- Internal control:		
E. Performed patient test	**S**	**U**
1.		
2.		
3.		
4.		
POSITIVE seen as: NEGATIVE seen as: INVALID seen as:		
*Accurate Results _____ Instructor Confirmation _____		

Appendix: Forms for Documenting Safety, Quality Assurance

Follow-up: Postanalytical Phase	Scores	
	S	U
*F. Proper documentation		
1. On control/patient log: _____ yes _____ no		
2. Documentation on patient chart (see below)		
3. Identified "critical values" and took appropriate steps to notify physician. EXPECTED VALUES FOR ANALYTE:		
G. Proper disposal and disinfection		
1. Disposed of all sharps into biohazard sharps containers.		
2. Disposed of all other regulated medical waste into biohazard bags.		
3. Disinfected test area and instruments according to OSHA guidelines.		
4. Sanitized hands after removing gloves.		
Column Totals		

Patient Name: _____

Patient Chart Entry: (Include when, what, how, why, any additional information, and the signature of the person charting.)

_____

_____

_____

SAMPLE HEALTH ASSESSMENT FORM

Please print clearly: Date _____

Name _____   Address _____

City _____   State _____   ZIP _____

Telephone _____   Age (date of birth) _____/_____/_____

Sex _____   Race _____   Ht. _____   Wt. _____

Do you consider yourself overweight? _____   If so, how much? _____

Name of family doctor _____   When last seen? _____

Do you smoke? _____   If yes, how many packs per day _____   Alcohol use? _____

Do you have   _____ Heart trouble   _____ High blood pressure

                       _____ Kidney problems   _____ Heart attack before/after 40

Are you taking medication for cholesterol? _____   Blood pressure? _____   Other? _____

Do you exercise regularly? _____   When did you last eat? _____ hours

---

When you are finished with all your tests, please return to this room for final review of your results.

RELEASE:

I release _____ and the Health Technology Students from any liability as a result of my participation in this free Health Fair.

Signature _____   Date _____

Parent/Guardian _____   Witness _____

TEST	NORMAL LIMITS	RESULTS	FURTHER EVALUATION _____

URINALYSIS   ☐

Glucose	NEG	
Bilirubin	NEG	
Ketone	NEG	
Spec grav	1.005–1.030	
Blood	NEG	
pH	6.0–8.0	
Protein	NEG/TRACE	
Urobil.	NORM	
Nitrite	NEG	
Leukocytes	NEG	

Clinitek: asterisk (*) indicates further evaluation

Urinalysis

Routine urinalysis is a basic test, but it provides the physician with a tremendous amount of information about a disease. This test can help confirm or rule out a suspected diagnosis. It is a routine test that is repeated annually or as frequently as necessary to evaluate the patient's health status.

HEMATOLOGY

Anemia   Hemoglobin: >12 g/dL   _____   ☐

Hematocrit: >32%   _____   ☐

Anemia Check

The hemoglobin and hematocrit tests determine the oxygen-carrying ability of the blood. They are simple and efficient methods to detect any anemia. A patient is considered anemic if the hemoglobin value is < 12 g/dL or the hematocrit is < 34%. Low values are caused by hemorrhage, pregnancy, recent menstruation, iron deficiency, or other conditions that the physician needs to evaluate.

Erythrocyte Sedimentation Rate (ESR) = 0–20 mm/hr _____   ☐

Erythrocyte sedimentation rates are increased in infectious and inflammatory diseases, tissue destruction, and other conditions that increase the plasma fibrinogen level.

COAGULATION

INRatio   _____ INR

ProTime   _____ seconds

> Desirable <u>0.8–1.2</u> INR
>
> Therapeutic <u>1.5–4.0</u> INR
>
> PT = _____ seconds

BLOOD CHEMISTRY

Glucose

    Fasting _____ (8 or more hours since eating)

    Random (hours since eating) _____ hr

    Normal 80–125 (if 2 hr after eating) _____

Hemoglobin A$_{1c}$ **Desirable levels are < 7%**   **Result** _____

WARNING SIGNS OF DIABETES	
Type 1 Diabetes	Type 2 Diabetes
Constant urination Abnormal thirst Unusual hunger Rapid loss of weight Irritability Obvious weakness or fatigue Nausea and vomiting	Drowsiness Itching A family history of diabetes Blurred vision Excessive weight Tingling, numbness in feet Easy fatigue Skin infections and slow healing

LIPID PROFILE (CHOLESTECH TEST)

Lipid Profile	Desirable Numbers	Cholestech Results
Total cholesterol	< 200 mg/dL	
HDL cholesterol	> 40 mg/dL	
LDL cholesterol	< 130 mg/dL	
Triglycerides	< 150 mg/dL	
TC/HDL ratio	4.5 or less	
Glucose	Fasting: 60-110 mg/dL	
	Nonfasting: < 160 mg/dL	

Cholesterol

Cholesterol measurements are used to diagnose and monitor disorders involving excess cholesterol in the blood and fat metabolism disorders. These conditions often are associated with coronary heart disease. It is thought that lowering mean cholesterol levels can reduce coronary heart disease.

CHEMISTRY PROFILE I-STAT (Chem 81)

Test	Test Symbol	Units	Reference Range	Result
Sodium	Na	mmol/L	138–146	
Potassium	K	mmol/L	3.5–4.9	
Chloride	Cl	mmol/L	98–109	
Total carbon dioxide	TCO_2	mmol/L	24–29	
Ionized calcium	iCa	mmol/L	1.12–1.32	
Glucose	Glu	mg/dL	70–105	
Urea nitrogen	BUN	mg/dL	8–26	
Creatinine	Crea	mg/dL	0.6–1.3	
Hematocrit	Hct	% PCV	38–51	
Hemoglobin*	Hb	g/dL	12–17	
Anion gap*	AnGap	mmol/L	10–20	

* These results are figured mathematically from the other results (not directly).

FECAL OCCULT BLOOD

Results: Positive _____ Negative _____

ECG AND SPIROMETRY: See attached reports.

REVIEW OF ALL RESULTS:

Appendix: Forms for Documenting Safety, Quality Assurance

PROFESSIONAL EVALUATION FORM FOR THE LABORATORY CLASSROOM

Student: _____

Class: _____

Date: _____

Semester: _____

Number of Hours Absent: _____

Number of Tardies: _____

Objective	Very Satisfactory 3	Satisfactory 2	Unsatisfactory 1	Comments
Exhibits professional written communication (e.g., appearance, language, grammar)				
Uses the class materials appropriately (e.g., equipment, supplies, computers, cleanup)				
Provides instructor with all necessary information in a timely and organized manner (e.g., meets due dates, make-ups turned in within a week)				
Adheres to specific course policies (e.g., make-up guidelines, skill check-offs, externship guidelines)				
Projects a positive attitude and motivation (e.g., seen during lectures and labs)				
Displays professional verbal communication at all times (e.g., respectful, tactful)				
Maintains confidentiality of all personal interactions at all times (see rules of confidentiality in handbook)				
Projects professional work ethics (e.g., responsible, accountable, independent, full use of laboratory time: practice, study, computer)				
Cooperates with fellow students (e.g., team projects, skill practice, study groups)				
Displays responsible attendance behavior (e.g., arriving on time, calling in if detained or absent, prepared for next class session)				
Dresses appropriately (see handbook)				

Additional Comments: _____

_____

_____

Student Signature _____

Instructor _____

Appendix: Forms for Documenting Safety, Quality Assurance